DRUGS
OF
ABUSE

Second Edition

A. JAMES GIANNINI, M.D.

Clinical Professor, Department of Psychiatry
Ohio State University
Columbus, Ohio

Corporate Medical Director
Chemical Abuse Centers, Inc.
Austintown, Canton, Columbus — Ohio

Practice Management Information Corporation
Los Angeles, California

Library of Congress Cataloging-in-Publication Data

Giannini, A. James, 1947-
   Drugs of abuse / A. James Giannini ; contributing authors, Ned
   Underwood, Nancy Luskovac. -- 2nd ed.
      p. cm.
   Includes bibliographical references.
   ISBN 1-57066-053-0
   1. Drug abuse. 2. Drugs of abuse. 3. Neuropsychopharmacology.
   I. Title
   [DNLM: 1. Substance Abuse. 2. Drugs. WM 270 G433d 1996]
   RC564.D787 1996
   616.86--DC20
   DNLM/DLC
   for Library of Congress   96-24680
                                                                  CIP

ISBN: 1-57066-053-0

Printed in the United States of America

Practice Management Information Corp. (PMIC)
4727 Wilshire Blvd., Suite 300
Los Angeles, CA 90010
1-800/MED-SHOP
internet: medicalbookstore.com

ABOUT THE AUTHOR

A. James Giannini, M.D., is a biological psychiatrist specializing in drug abuse. He graduated with honors in psychiatry from the University of Pittsburgh and received his psychiatric training at Yale University where he was chief resident.

Dr. Giannini is currently diplomate candidate at the University of London in the United Kingdom. He is a former professor and vice chairman of psychiatry at Northeastern Ohio University's College of Medicine and is clinical professor of psychiatry at Ohio State University. He has served as chairman of the National Advisory Commission on Rape at the National Institute of Mental Health, and has worked as an American Participant in the field of drug abuse for the United States Information Agency in Europe, the Middle East and Caribbean.

Dr. Giannini has been elected Fellow of the American Psychiatric Association, the American College of Clinical Pharmacology, and The Royal Society of Medicine (Great Britain).

He has received many awards for his work, including the Bronze Award from the British Medical Association, the Silver Rose Award from the Associazone Italiana Donnadori d'Organo. He is also listed in *The Best Doctors in America.*

Dr. Giannini has written 8 books and 250 articles in the area of biological psychiatry and chemical dependence. He also serves as corporate medical director of Chemical Abuse Centers, Inc., an innovative treatment program whose concepts have been adapted for use in Italy, Cyprus, St. Lucia, Barbados, Slovenia, Macedonia, Montenegro, and Croatia.

CONTRIBUTING AUTHORS

Ned Underwood, D.O.
Youngstown, Ohio
* *Professor of Internal Medicine,*
  Ohio University
* *Chairman, Department of Internal Medicine,*
  Youngstown Osteopathic Hospital

Senior Author

Chapter 16: Cardiovascular Complications of Drug Abuse

Nancy Leskovac
Austintown, Ohio
* *Nutritionist*
  Chemical Abuse Centers, Inc.

Junior Author

Chapter 19: Nutritional Aspects of Drug Abuse

DISCLAIMER

This publication is designed to offer basic and practical information on drugs of abuse. The information presented is based on the experience and interpretation of the author. Although the information has been carefully researched and checked for accuracy, currency and completeness, neither the author nor the publisher accept any responsibility or liability with regard to errors, omissions, misuse or misinterpretation.

DEDICATION

This book is dedicated to my daughters Jocelyn Danielle Giannini and Juliette Nicole Giannini, and their friends from Bassett Hall: Lady Bosworth Fields, Lord Trelayne Trafalgar; Sir Watkins Agincourt and the late Squire Hastings of Meander.

TABLE OF CONTENTS

PREFACE

Drugs of Abuse, Second Edition, is a compendium drawn from journals from all scientific fields which affect chemical dependency. This volume carefully describes the basis of the addictive properties of each drug and then leads the reader through the assessment, detoxification and treatment phases. The "typical case presentation" provided in each chapter is a unique teaching tool by which the clinician can study the application of his or her knowledge.

Chapters on legal and organizational issues make this a valuable resource for the administrator. Clinicians will appreciate the chapters discussing co-existing psychiatric, eating and nutritional disorders. There is also a useful chapter on the nursing or pregnant addict.

This book is a highly personal product. As those readers familiar with Dr. Giannini's work will note, there are richly detailed perspectives from a variety of non-traditional areas. These are drawn from artistic, cultural, literary, anthropological and historical sources, and will deepen the clinician's understanding beyond a narrow technological base. The first edition of *Drugs of Abuse* was a major reference work. I predict that this second edition will prove to be a classic.

Carlton Turner, Ph.D., D. Sc.

Dr. Turner is currently President and CEO of Carrington Laboratories in Irving, Texas. Previously he served as Director of the President's Drug Abuse Policy Office during the Reagan Administration.

ACKNOWLEDGEMENTS

The author wishes to thank those individuals who directly and indirectly assisted in the production of *Drugs of Abuse*, Second Edition. Gratitude is extended to Marian Fry and her assistants Jenny Mrgan and Donna Riley for word processing the original manuscript, and to Amy Dyer for research assistance.

INTRODUCTION

The recent Robert Wood Johnson Foundation report on the nation's number-one health problem set out the challenges that face all physicians and public health officials. The United States spends a staggering $238 billion in unnecessary costs annually because of substance abuse.

Alcohol, tobacco, and illicit drugs are major causes of morbidity and mortality. They are responsible for premature deaths, accidents, fires, motor vehicle deaths, drowning, assaults, family and psychological problems, and numerous life-shortening medical problems.

The American Medical Association estimates that 25 to 40 percent of patients in general hospital beds are being treated for complications of alcohol abuse alone.[1] Alcohol is the major cause of cirrhosis, which is the ninth-leading cause of death. Traffic crashes are the single greatest cause of death among young Americans, and the use of drugs and alcohol contributes to the majority of these. On average, people dying from alcohol-related causes lose 26 years from their normal life expectancy.

Illicit drugs are clearly related to premature disability and death, HIV/AIDS, child abuse and neglect, trauma, accidental deaths, homicides, violent crime, medical and psychiatric problems. A startling 375,000 babies are born each year who have been exposed to illicit drugs in utero.

While it is difficult to know the exact costs to our society even in simple measures like dollars, the RWJ report approximates alcohol costs at $98.6 billion, drug costs at $66.9 billion and tobacco costs exceeding $72 billion annually. These calculations include direct medical costs, lost productivity, injury, illness, premature death, as well as costs due to crime, motor vehicle accidents, incarceration and fetal alcohol syndrome. Just looking at unnecessary healthcare costs, alcohol abuse alone costs $10.5 billion per year and drug abuse $3.2 billion annually.

Physicians are prime opinion leaders. As experts in their field, physicians have a special role in influencing standards and expectations. They will be vital to any attempt to reduce drug use and dependence. This book is a great tool to that end. Physician education and practice are rarely consonant with the occurrence and significance of societal alcohol and other drug dependence. In *Drugs of Abuse*, the authors take physicians through this learning process with tremendous understanding and skill.

Physicians are doing a better job of taking a nicotine, alcohol and drug history and then asking the patient to quit using these substances. Still, physicians do not generally understand what can be done to improve the success rate of diagnosis, detoxification and abstinence. Physicians have an important role in early detection and initiation of treatment. Yet most miss important opportunities to make an early diagnosis and begin medical intervention and treatment. As the authors recognize, treatment of addiction begins with an early and accurate diagnosis.

Many times a physician's medical education leaves him or her without answers to questions such as, what is the difference between drinking and being an alcoholic? The medical approach to addiction taken in this book correctly takes into account the heterogeneity of abuse and addiction symptomatology in a context of a core syndrome. Identified risk factors such as *in utero* exposure, psychopathology and family history, are becoming important as science develops a new understanding of addiction liability on the basis of brain reinforcement and pathological attachment.

The psychiatric physician needs to incorporate this comprehensive approach with extensive clinical experience to improve detection and outcomes. Addicts complicate their diagnosis by minimizing their drug use and drinking, by denying problems, by emphasizing their depression, and by generally preferring to be diagnosed as a psychiatric patient and not a drug addict or alcoholic.

This new edition of *Drugs of Abuse* helps doctors understand that, common to most definitions of dependence are: (1) the compulsion to use the drug with loss of control despite guilt; and (2) thoughts about limiting the use of the drug and a subsequent withdrawal or abstinence syndrome of varying intensity.

Addiction has two central features. The first is loss of control over the use of an addicting substances. This is characterized by continued use despite adverse consequences of that use (the unmanageability of substance use and therefore of life itself). The second central feature of addiction is denial of the use of alcohol and/or other intoxicating drugs, as well as the denial of the consequences of that use (i.e., dishonesty).

The most intuitively satisfying laboratory model for addiction is voluntary self-administration or lever pressing, first described by B.F. Skinner. Alcohol and other drugs stimulate their own taking. Addicts become attached to alcohol or drugs, and also to their liquor store or drug sources, as well as to the friends with whom they drink or use drugs. In addition to craving the rewarding aspects of the drug, addicts establish conditioned attachments that potentiate the impact of other drugs and reinforcers. These are incentive-motivational or priming effects, such as the association of the crack pipe with cocaine euphoria, or salted peanuts with an alcohol buzz, or the smell of the cork before drinking wine.

In thinking about treatments to reverse the mechanisms driving addictive behavior, it is useful to distinguish between positive reinforcement and negative reinforcement. Positive reinforcement involves the euphoria and very strong good feelings associated with drinking or drug taking. Negative reinforcement involves both the removal of distress and the actual negative effect or discomfort of withdrawal.

Most addicted people report that both positive and negative reinforcement play important roles in initiating and maintaining addictive alcohol and other drug use. However, withdrawal distress or even cravings are rarely causes of relapse; untreated co-morbid disorders and unmanaged drives for the drug are. Physicians, by treating withdrawal, are treating negative reinforcement without attention to the drive for positive brain reinforcement.

Positive reinforcement is more likely to be mentioned earlier in the addict's career and most likely related to the pathological attachment between the addict and the drug. It is remarkable that drug-taking persists when addicts clearly describe that alcohol does not make them high anymore; that they have lost their job, their home, their health and their loved ones. But since drug-taking stimulates itself and establishes a strong new drive state, such an absence of true euphoria may be another example of how behavior talks louder than words.

This book summarizes what I call the three general phases to the treatment of addiction. The first is Getting Started, the process of developing the willingness to enter treatment, or what Alcoholics Anonymous calls "the desire" to stop drinking and using drugs. There are many important roles in this first phase of the addiction treatment experience. These include decreasing social tolerance for the use of alcohol and other drugs, via drug testing in the workplace or stricter prohibitions on driving while impaired (DWI). The modern structured intervention is an organized approach to overcoming the most basic stage of denial in order to get addicted people into treatment.

The second phase of addiction treatment is stopping use, which can be done either on an inpatient or an outpatient basis. It is in this stage that medical treatment of abstinence may be important. This is where organized, medically managed detoxification takes place.

The third phase of addiction treatment is staying clean and sober. This is where relapse prevention and the 12-step programs of Alcoholics Anonymous, Narcotics Anonymous, Al-Anon, and other organizations built on the original foundations of AA, play their biggest roles. Relapse-preventing psychopharmacology is an important new addition to this phase. Using medications like the opiate antagonist naltrexone, which denies brain-reward access to drugs, rather than punishing the addict for using the drug, is now in widespread use and helping to promote dramatic changes in the field of Addiction Medicine and Addiction Psychiatry. Treatment with naltrexone has made some relapsing— and even chronically relapsing—alcoholics more amenable to 12-step fellowships and behavior change. Rather than an either-or-approach, current treatment of the addict with depression (or other major co-morbid psychiatric or medical illness) involves vigorous treatment of all disorders.

A desirable treatment outcome over a period of many years was virtually unheard of following decades of repeated detoxification. The medical profession was nevertheless slow to recognize the implications of this observation. Rather than question underlying assumptions which placed medical skills essential in the diagnoses and treatment of withdrawal at the center of the problem of addiction treatment, physicians seemed content to recycle addicted people through one emergency room or detoxification experience after another. Drugs of Abuse helps to rectify this problem by dealing with all aspects of addiction.

Mark S. Gold, M.D.
Professor, University of Florida Brain Institute
Departments of Neuroscience, Psychiatry, Community Health
and Family Medicine, Gainesville, Florida

NOTES

1. American Medical Association. *Factors Contributing to the Health Care Cost Problem.* Chicago, IL: American Medical Association, 1993.

CHAPTER 1

MEDICAL MODELS OF ADDICTION

In 1964, neuroscientist Aryeh Routtenberg implanted electrodes into the brains of laboratory rats, placing them so that the current would activate the pleasure centers. The rats were then given a choice of two levers: one lever controlled the food supply and the second controlled the electrical current. No rat had difficulty making a choice. Every single one was too intent on maintaining the current to stop for food. As a result, each animal blissfully died of starvation.[1]

Just as electricity substituted for food as a primary drive in this experiment, so do the drugs of addiction. An addictive drug must by definition be pleasurable. The derived pleasure can then become so intense as to displace the primary drives of water, food and sex.[2] The chemical interaction between drugs and the synaptic receptors in the brain thus makes up the neurochemical pathology that produces addiction, a pseudodrive albeit a powerful one.[3]

Opiate addiction has been demonstrated to be related to norepinephrine and beta-endorphin, whereas barbiturate and benzodiazepine addictions are thought to be caused by the effects of gamma-aminobutyric acid (GABA). Likewise, cocaine addiction has been reported to be a function of noradrenergic and dopaminergic transmission. GABA depletion and abnormalities of G-protein are seen in alcohol addiction. Finally, phencyclidine manifests quite complex actions at multiple receptor sites.

The medical model of addiction is based on the assumption that a substance such as cocaine or heroin interacts with a susceptible host. The host's susceptibility is due to a genetic predisposition to initiate the disease process.[4] The diagnostic criterion for addiction involves an impairment of lifestyle. The addict is obsessed with the acquisition of the particular drug and is compulsive regarding its use. The obsessions, compulsions and persistent relapses utilizing a specific drug then preclude interpersonal relationships and normal function. Like the role of electricity in Routtenberg's rats, the use of an addicting drug becomes a pseudodrive displacing the primary drives of food, water and sex. All other aspects of the addict's life become peripheral.[2]

Since different drugs inhibit or stimulate the release of different neurotransmitters to produce their effects, specific drug addiction and abuse is often misdiagnosed due to the multiple signs and symptoms associated with each separate drug. The proper use of the medical model can assist in the accurate diagnosis and efficient treatment of drug abuse. In mastering the medical model, only a few principles must be learned. These can then be applied to most drug abuse situations. The medical model thus eliminates the need to memorize the hundreds of symptoms and dozens of treatment modalities that are otherwise required to sufficiently attend to a drug-addicted population.[4]

This model is based in part upon the biopsychiatric principle that drugs of abuse do not interact uniquely with the brain to produce highly specific symptoms. Rather, these drugs either stimulate or inhibit the rate of release of a limited number of neurotransmitters. Six neurotransmitters—acetylcholine, beta-endorphin, dopamine, gamma-aminobutyric acid, norepinephrine and serotonin—account for most of the symptoms seen in the mood- and thought-altering drugs commonly abused in the United States. By mastering a basic knowledge of neurotransmitters, physicians can expeditiously recognize the specific drug being abused. Once the type of drug is diagnosed, treatment then logically follows. The treatment protocol is thereupon based upon alterations in specific neurotransmitter activity.[5]

ACETYLCHOLINE

Most acetylcholine activity is generated by gating potassium channels. Acetylcholine is distributed in the nucleus basalis of Meynert and the nigrostriatal tract. Degeneration of the nucleus basalis causes degeneration of projecting cholinergic neurons to the cerebral cortex. This produces the intellectual alterations seen in anticholinergic delirium. In fact, degeneration of acetylcholine tracts is consistently noted in Alzheimer's disease.

There is a second action in the nigrostriatal tract where acetylcholine maintains a rough equilibrium with dopamine. A relative increase in acetylcholine levels in the tract can produce primary or secondary Parkinsonism. A third area of acetylcholine activity is in the reticular activating substance (RAS) which maintains the waking state. The RAS is also the entry point of new memories.

There are two basic types of acetylcholine receptors: the muscarinic and the nicotinic. Muscarinic receptors are predominantly central in distribution whereas nicotinic receptors are usually peripheral. Stimulation of central muscarinic receptors can cause spasticity or tremors due to activation of basal ganglia. Blockade can reduce memory formation due to decreased activity at the RAS. Peripherally, muscarinic receptor-activity can inhibit cardiac activity and stimulate gastrointestinal tract motility.

The peripheral activity at nicotinic receptors is generally dichotomous. Small doses of compounds with nicotinic activity stimulate release of epinephrine from the adrenal medulla; higher doses inhibit release via splanchnic nerve stimulation. Likewise, low concentrations will stimulate the autonomic ganglia and myoneural junctions but higher concentrations will suppress activity by blockade in these two areas. Nicotinic sites also activate chemoreceptors in the carotid body; thermal receptors in the skin and tongue; and pressure/stretch receptors in the skin, tongue and gastrointestinal tract. Centrally, excitation produces tremors via the basal ganglia and respiratory depression via the medulla oblongata.

DOPAMINE

Dopamine is a major catecholamine neurotransmitter. This transmitter stimulates both mood and thought by the stimulation of adenylate cyclase. Low levels of dopamine are associated with depression whereas high levels are found in psychotic disorders such as schizophrenia and chorea. Degeneration of dopaminergic neurons in the nigrostriatal tract is seen in primary Parkinson's disease whereas inhibition of dopaminergic neurons is seen in secondary Parkinsonism (vide supra).

Centrally, dopamine is the primary pathway between the nucleus accumbens and the pars compacta which function as pleasure centers in humans. Dopamine also inhibits prolactin release from the pituitary gland via the tuberoinfundibular pathway. In this manner, substances which inhibit dopamine increase levels of prolactin. Peripherally, dopamine receptors have a direct inotropic effect on the heart, i.e., there is increased cardiac output without appreciable change in heart rate or blood pressure. Vascular effects include vasodilatation resulting in decreased flow-resistance. As a result, renal blood flow, glomerular filtration rate and sodium excretion are, in cascade fashion, enhanced.

BETA-ENDORPHIN

Beta-endorphin (β-endorphin) is an opiate derived from beta-lipoprotein. It is located at many sites within the brain, including the nucleus locus ceruleus, hippocampus, nucleus solitarius, substantia gelatinosa and thalamus. Subjectively, beta-endorphin produces euphoria, a sense of well-being and bodywide analgesia. It can also function in the nucleus locus ceruleus to inhibit norepinephrine release. Evidence also exists that beta-endorphin inhibits serotonin release in the pontine raphe nuclei.[6] In general, beta-endorphin activity is usually inhibitory, except for excitatory actions at the hippocampal pyramids and Renshaw cells. Inhibition is due to over-stimulation of the cyclic nucleotide, guanylate cyclase. This produces hyperpolarization at any and all neuron types.

GABA

Gamma-aminobutyric (γ-aminobutyric) acid, or GABA, is distributed throughout the brain and accounts for over 30 percent of all receptor sites there. The highest levels are found in the substantia nigra, limbic system, and globus pallidus. Unlike other neurotransmitters seen in drugs of abuse, its actions are exclusively inhibitory. It is the major inhibitory neurotransmitter of the brain and one of two major inhibitory transmitters in the spinal cord. GABA acts by gating chloride channels. Like beta-endorphin, it produces a hyperpolarization. This diminishes the generation of an action potential in post-synaptic neurons, inhibiting neuronal firing.[7]

GABA has two types of receptors—direct and indirect. Sedative hypnotics act directly on the chloride channel via the B-P (i.e., barbiturate-picrotoxin) receptors. Benzodiazepines exert only an indirect action on this channel. They act at the B-Z (i.e., benzodiazepine) receptors to enhance GABA activity.

NOREPINEPHRINE

Norepinephrine is a stimulatory neurotransmitter. It is synthesized from dopamine. Its release is inhibited by beta-endorphin and high levels of serotonin. Centrally, high concentrations are found in the nucleus locus ceruleus, a paired nucleus located in the pons near the third ventricle.

Norepinephrine is a catecholamine which generally regulates mood. While low levels of norepinephrine are associated with depression, high levels are associated with mania and anxiety. Centrally, norepinephrine also maintains a sleeping state. Peripherally, norepinephrine is manufactured in the adrenal glands and has vasoconstrictive activity. It raises free fatty acid levels by activating triglyceride lipase.

SEROTONIN

Serotonin is an indolamine which is located in the five paired pontine raphe nuclei. Serotonin is a stimulant and may inhibit norepinephrine production. It is associated with initiating sleep and maintaining the rapid eye movement (REM) phase of sleep.

Low levels of serotonin are associated with depression while essentially high levels are associated with psychoses. High levels of peripheral serotonin, as in carcinoid, can produce flushing, gastrointestinal hypermotility, cramping and destruction of cardiac valvular connective tissue.

ACTIVITY OF DRUGS OF ABUSE

The actions of the drugs of abuse are based on their stimulation or retardation of blockade of neurotransmitter release and/or receptor sites associated with a specific neurotransmitter (see Table 1-1).

The GABA-minergic drugs — including alcohol, barbiturates, ethchlorvynol, glutethimide, meprobamate, and the benzodiazepines — all suppress neuronal function by activating the GABA receptors. As a result, there is a slowing and eventual paralysis of sensory and motor function in the central nervous system. These physiological effects are expressed systematically by confusion, sedation, slowing of consciousness and coma. This occurs as a result of the relative slowing of the release of stimulatory transmitters (e.g., norepinephrine, serotonin, dopamine) by increased GABA release. In addition to such peripheral effects, there is bradycardia, bradypnea and hypotension. Bradypnea may proceed to acidosis and bradycardia to arrhythmias.

Table 1-1: Neurotransmitter Action

Neurotransmitter	Central Action	Central Location	Interacting Drugs
Acetylcholine	Counter balance dopamine; initiate short-term memory	Caudate nucleus Lentiform nucleus Cerebral cortex Nucleus basalis of Meynert Nigrostriatal tract Reticular activating substance	Anticholinergics Phencyclidine
GABA	General inhibition of other neuro-transmitters	Throughout brain	Alcohol Benzodiazepines Chloral hydrate Marijuana Phencyclidine Sedative hypnotics Volatiles
Beta-Endorphin	Modulates mood; modulates pain perception; inhibits norepinephrine release	Thalamus Arcuate and pre- mammillary nuclei Hippocampus Nucleus locus ceruleus Nucleus solitarius Substantia gelatinosa	Marijuana Opiates Phencyclidine
Dopamine	Counterbalances acetylcholine; stimulates pleasure centers; modulates mood; affects intellectual processes; inhibits prolactin release	Caudate nucleus Lentiform nucleus Nucleus accumbens Tuberoinfundibular pathway Nigrostriatal tract	Cocaine Khat Marijuana Phencyclidine Steroids Sympathomimetics Volatiles
Norepinephrine	Modulates mood; Maintains sleep state	Nucleus locus ceruleus Pontine/medullary cell groups	Cocaine Khat Marijuana Opiates Phencyclidine Sympathomimetics

Neurotransmitter	Central Action	Central Location	Interacting Drugs
Serotonin	Modulates mood and anxiety; inhibits norepinephrine release; initiates sleep cycle; involved in REM sleep; involved in anxiety and despair	Pontine raphe nuclei	Marijuana Phencyclidine Psychedelics

As endogenous substances (such as alcohol or barbiturates) stimulate GABA-minergic function, the brain parsimoniously reduces the rate of GABA production. As a result, the supply of endogenous GABA is progressively decreased.

If the GABA-minergic drug is suddenly withdrawn, the inhibitory actions of the GABA system are reduced since there is little endogenous GABA to compensate for the sudden withdrawal of the drugs. As a result, there is a rebound of excitatory neurotransmitters previously under GABA control.

As serotonin and norepinephrine rebound, there is hyper-alertness, hyperglycemia, hypertension, hyperreflexia, and pupillary dilation. Dopamine rebound is associated with tremors, hallucinations, delusions and seizures. Increased activity levels of acetylcholine may lead to hypothermia and flushing.

GABA-minergic withdrawal is treated directly. While rebound of dopamine, norepinephrine and serotonin produce the pathological consequences, the primary etiology nevertheless occurs at GABA-minergic sites. Therefore, in the case of direct acting drugs such as barbiturate, glutethimide and methaqualone, a direct acting GABA-minergic drug is substituted. Gradually this drug, such as a barbiturate, is withdrawn over time so that the body can adapt to a progressive withdrawal.

With slow downward titration of dosage, GABA-minergic systems can gradually recover and reactivate. In the case of indirect GABA-minergic drugs such as alcohol, benzodiazepines, chloral hydrate and paraldehyde, an indirect GABA-minergic agent such as a benzodiazepine is used. In similar fashion, as the dosage is titrated downward, the GABA-minergic system gradually reactivates.

Opiates act on the nucleus accumbens to produce their effects. However, withdrawal symptoms are mediated through the locus ceruleus. A specific type of opiate receptor, the μ-receptor, regulates the release of norepinephrine. During intoxication or addiction, there is a suppression of norepinephrine release. During withdrawal, the opiate suppression is terminated and there is a massive rebound release of norepinephrine. Since norepinephrine is a stimulant, thereby results the typical response of noradrenergic stimulation: muscular cramping, tachycardia and flushing.

Sympathomimetics cause a release of stored or new dopamine from the presynaptic vessels. This effect is seen in amphetamine; in more central-acting amphetamine derivatives such as methamphetamine; and in hallucinatory derivatives such as methylene-dioxy-methamphetamine. (Cocaine, although it is discussed in a separate chapter, is a sympathomimetic.)

The sympathomimetics increase the rate of release of both dopamine and norepinephrine while reducing the rate of deaminase reuptake. As a result, large amounts of these two stimulatory amines are permitted to remain in the synaptic cleft for longer periods of time. This creates a doubly enhanced stimulatory effect. In this case, less deaminase reuptake occurs intraneuronally and more norepinephrine and dopamine are degraded extraneuronally in the synaptic cleft by catechol-O-methyltransferase (COMT). The resulting metabolite, 5-OH-tyramine, is not recycled. Over time, the amounts of available norepinephrine and dopamine are reduced. Therefore, the degree of stimulatory "rush" or "high" is gradually and progressively attenuated as the raw material (i.e., the dopamine and norepinephrine creating this rush) is reduced. Tolerance thereby occurs.

These rushes produce a progressively decreased peripheral stimulatory effect such as tachycardia, vasoconstriction and pupillary dilation. Central effects including the resultant anorexia, euphoria, hypervigilance, increased level of endurance and activity, hypersexuality and grandiosity are also reduced in intensity.

Because the supply of norepinephrine and dopamine is progressively reduced, the body must always play catch-up. Using ever-larger doses of a stimulatory enables the drug addict to catch the high that was obtained in the previous dose. However, when the drug ration is cut off, the relatively small supply of remaining dopamine and norepinephrine can no longer produce even a maintenance state. Withdrawal then results.

Symptomatically this presents as muscle cramping, hypersomnia, extreme hunger and a profound dysphoria.

Psychedelic agents act by exciting presynaptic serotonergic receptors in the pontine raphe nuclei. As a result, there is a temporary disruption of vision, proprioception and perception. There is a blending of senses (for example "hearing a cinnamon color") and REM-like changes in the EEG which produces a dream-like quality for the abusers. Actions on the pontine raphe nuclei produce distortions; stimulation of the auditory and visual centers produce hallucinations. Actions of the hippocampus, hypothalamus and amygdala alter the transfer and integration of sensory messages.

Prolonged use of psychedelics deplete the supply of serotonin and may lead to depression. While no known agent is able to reverse the effects of a psychedelic hallucination, heterocyclic serotonergic antidepressants such as fluoxetine are useful in treating the dysphoria associated with prolonged psychedelic use.

Anticholinergic drugs — including naturally occurring botanicals such as asthmador, wolfsbane and jimson weed, as well as over-the-counter and prescription medications such as diphenhydramine and benztropine — block activity of acetylcholine. In low doses, this produces a subjective feeling of relaxation, pleasant fatigue and somnolence. High doses can result in visual and tactile hallucinations. The tranquilizing effect results from an overbalancing of dopamine in the nigrostriatal tract and peripheral blockade of autonomic ganglia and myoneural junctions.

At higher doses there is decreased blockade of activity in the reticular activating substance so that there is difficulty in receiving and processing new concepts. Acetylcholinergic antagonism at projections from the nucleus basalis of Meynert to the neocortex results in disruption of intellectual organization and, over time, frank psychosis.

The dissociatives act at all the neurotransmitter sites discussed above. The actions of the dissociatives such as phencyclidine (PCP) or phenylhexylpyrrolidine (PHP) mimic the catecholaminergic stimulatory effects of cocaine and amphetamine; the psychedelic effects of LSD by its stimulatory actions of serotonin; and the anticholinergic effects of atropine and asthmador by inhibition of acetylcholine. Its opiate actions are complex, including simultaneous stimulation and inhibition of opiate release. GABA-minergic action may also be as ambivalently complex.

Table 1-2: Drug Specific Interventions

Drug Class	Effects	Treatment
Sedative/ Tranquilizers	Diminished activity of GABA inhibition	Gradually taper the sedative/hypnotic. Substitute phenobarbital or chlordiazepoxide (Librium, Lipoxide, Mitran, etc.) depending upon the drug of abuse, to allow restoration of GABA activity.
Stimulants	Depletion of dopamine and norepinephrine	Administer bromocriptine (Parlodel), a dopamine agonist, to detoxify. Administer desipramine (Norpramin, Pertofrane) to enhance norepinephrine receptors to decrease cravings.
Opiates	Norepinephrine release	Administer naloxone (Narcan) to reverse acute intoxication and overdose. Administer clonidone (Catapres) to block norepinephrine release to detoxify. Administer naltrexone (Trexan), an opiate antagonist, for long-term maintenance.
Psychedelic agents	Enhance serotonin activity	Place patient in a quiet environment to allow the effects of the drug to wear off. Administer lorazepam (Alzapam, Ativan), an indirect GABA agonist that blocks serotonin effects, to prevent panic.
Dissociatives	Stimulation of dopamine and norepinephrine receptors and blockage of acetylcholine	Administer haloperidol (Haldol), a dopamine-2 agonist, to treat psychosis and block drug action.

Because of cholinergic stimulatory actions, the dissociatives produce tachycardia, hypervigilance, decreased coordination, increased activity and sometimes anxiety. The anticholinergic effects, especially in the RAS, produce amnestic episodes and confused thinking. By activating opiate receptors, the pain tolerance is dramatically increased and the patient intoxicated with a dissociative may appear to have superhuman strength due to the otherwise intolerable strains to which they subject their musculoskeletal system. The hot dry skin seen in the dissociative patient is due to the combination of peripheral serotonergic and peripheral anticholinergic activity.

Although a variety of systems are affected, the most clinically significant is dopaminergic. There is an activation of a DA-2 receptors in dissociative psychosis. Therefore, antidotal treatment involves the use of DA-2 blocker such as haloperidol or pimozide.

CONCLUSION

By carefully observing specific alterations on various bodily systems, the affected neurotransmitter(s) can be deduced. After determination of the specific transmitters, appropriate interventions can be instituted (Table 1-2). It should be noted, however, that pharmacological intervention treats only the symptoms associated with addiction and withdrawal.[8] While medico-pharmacological intervention emphasizes the passive role of the addicted patient, addiction requires initial repetitive voluntary use of the addicting drug.[9] Treating addicts requires intense rehabilitation after the detoxification takes place.

NOTES

1. High and hooked. The Economist 1993; **327**: 105-108.
2. Giannini AJ. Un modello biopsichiatrico per riconoseere la tossicomania. Ricerca e Salute 1990; **2(3)**: 4-11.
3. Miller NA, Giannini, AJ. The disease model of addiction. J Psychoactive Drugs 1990; **220(1)**: 83-85.
4. Shimada S, Kitayama S, et.al. Cloning and expression of a cocaine-sensitive dopamine transporter complementary DNA. Science 1991; **254(5031)**: 568-578.
5. Giannini AJ, Miller NA. Drug abuse: a biopsychiatric model. Am Fam Physician 1989; **40**: 173-182.
6. O'Brien CP. Self reinforcement model of opiate abstinence. Pharmacol Review 1976; **27**: 533-543.
7. Soyka M, Holzbach R, and Kuss HJ. Toxic delirium in alcoholic patients treated with antidepressants. Eur Addict Res 1994; **1**: 74-75.
8. Ticbout HM. Surrender versus compliance in therapy. Q J Stud Alc 1994; **14**: 58-68.

9. Miller NS. Drug addiction as a disease. In: NS Miller (Ed.), Comprehensive Handbook of Drug and Alcohol Addiction. NY: Marcel Dekker, 1991.

CHAPTER 2

ALCOHOL

Alcohol is the most ubiquitous of all drugs of abuse. Its range is worldwide. It has been manufactured since the dawn of history in every culture, range and climate. In fact, it is the only drug manufactured by animals other than man. Frank Buck documented orangutans in the jungles of Indonesia preparing and aging berrymash in the hollows of logs. The orangutans would then guard the berrymash on a periodic basis, returning weeks later to sample their fermented product.[1]

Although it is usually a legal product, alcohol is associated with numerous indirect deaths. These indirect deaths usually arise from industrial and highway accidents. It is directly responsible for cirrhosis, central nervous system degeneration and nutritional disorders which can lead to death or irreversible pathology.

Positively, alcohol products are used sacramentally in Christian and other rituals. Also, different forms of alcohol are agricultural mainstays in many regions of the world. It is one of the main pillars of the California economy as well as a major export product of France, Germany, Italy and Austria. Distilled alcoholic products have been integrated into the national cultures of many countries, such as the scotch of Scotland, the gin of England, the vodka of Russia, the schnapps of Germany, the sake of Japan and the bourbon of the United States.

The problem of alcohol lies not in the consequences of the drug itself but in the inability of the culture to integrate its use. Alcohol has devastated many aboriginal cultures. On the other hand, the people of the Italian Peninsula have made wine an integral part of their daily diet for nearly three millennia and have one of the lowest incidence of alcoholism and alcoholic-related disease in the world. Similar findings are noted also in Greece, Israel and Spain.

LABORATORY TESTING

Alcohol is a simple two-carbon molecule and can be easily tested in the laboratory. Generally, thin layer chromatography is not helpful. Most laboratories and many hospital emergency rooms use gas chromatography on a head-space sample.[2] This technique can distinguish between ethanol, methanol, isopropyl alcohol (isopropanol) and acetone. More sophisticated techniques are usually not necessary.

Because alcohol levels are generally employed for legal purposes, a chain-of-custody technique is mandatory. During this chain, it is necessary that the physician either draw the blood sample or witness it being drawn and then witness it being placed in the appropriate test tube or vial and sealed. In each case, every person who is involved in the extraction, storage and testing of the sample must sign a chain of custody form.[3]

BACKGROUND

All alcoholic beverages are produced by the action of yeast upon carbohydrates in plant products. When the yeast acts upon a simple sugar, wine is produced. Common sources of wine, in addition to grapes, include cherries, elderberries, blackberries and dandelions. Wines such as Marsala and Port may be fortified with additional alcohol. Carbonated wines such as champagne are referred to as "sparkling." All other wines are referred to as "still wines."

Beers are produced from the yeast fermentation of plant starches. Most of the world's beers are made from a combination of malted barley and hops in varying proportions.

Beers can be produced by using bottom-fermenting yeast, which sinks to the bottom of the vat after fermentation, or a top-fermenting yeast, which rises the surface as a result of carbon dioxide production. Most bottom fermented beers are "lager" beers. Common lagers include Dortmund, California steam, Munich and Pilsner. Popular top-fermented beers include porter and stout. Bock beer is a bottom-fermented nonlager beer found chiefly in the United States. Ale is any beer made solely from malted barley. Beers are also made from a variety of other products, including millet, sorghum, rye (kbass), rice (sake) or cactus (pulque).

Alcohol is the oldest of all recorded drugs. Alcoholic beverages are mentioned in the two oldest of mankind's books, the book of Genesis in the Bible, and the *Gilgamesh Epic*. In each of these books the subjects — Noah and Gilgamesh, respectively — become intoxicated.

Descriptions of wine production are found in pharaonic tombs in Egypt dating from 3000 B.C. Wine production then spread from Mesopotamian and Egyptian civilization throughout the Mediterranean. The Greeks created a god, Dionysus, under whose protection wine production was placed. Understanding the potent power of alcohol, their mythology included impairment of the judgement of the gods Mars and Zeus, as well as the massacre of Orpheus, all due to wine.

Drinking customs were described in Homer's *Iliad* and *Odyssey*. The Romans continued their worship of Dionysus, changing his name to Bacchus and placing a holiday of drunken revelry and sexual liberation, Bacchanalia, as his feast day. In the first century after Christ, Columella produced the first known treatise on viniculture, *De Re Rustica*.

Romans and Greeks used a variety of grapes to produce wine. However, since the Middle Ages, most wine produced in North America, South America and Europe has been a variety of *Vitis vinifera*.

Beer was first used by Bronze-Age Sumerians. Detailed instructions for producing beer were chronicled by the Roman emperor Marcus Aurelius who observed its manufacture by Germanic tribes. During the Medieval Era, Arab chemists discovered the process of distillation. It was introduced to Europe by monkish scholars and immediately adapted throughout the monasteries. The learned monks directly distilled various fermented plant juices or, alternatively, wines, producing a new type of alcoholic product called "liqueur."

Some of these liqueurs are still consumed today. Benedictine, produced by the Benedictine monks, remains popular. Others include chartreuse, rosolio, anisette, and Gemma d'Abetto. In Ireland, distillates of fermented barley were referred to as "usquebaugh," which loosely translated as "the water of life." From usquebaugh was derived the English word "whiskey."

In the 1600's, Francisca Sylvius distilled juniper berries while teaching medicine at the University of Leyden in the Netherlands. He used the French name of the juniper berry, "genievre," which was translated by the Dutch to "genever." During the religious wars of that century, the British soldiers readily adopted genever and brought it to England where its name was shortened to "gin." A far less expensive product than Scotch or Irish whiskey, it was immediately adopted by the lower classes. Because of the growth of cheap bars — which were literally "holes in the wall" where gin was poured through a knot-hole into the awaiting drinker's glass — the term "gin lane" entered our language to describe an area of squalor and deprivation.

In the eighteenth century, American farmers, unable to transport their corn (maize) to market before spoilage, began distilling this grain to produce bourbon and sour mash whiskey.

Another form of distillate includes tinctures or infusions. The first tincture was produced by Paracelsus, a German Renaissance medical professor. His product was laudanum, a tincture of opium, which remained popular through the nineteenth century. Its use died out, although it has enjoyed a "New Age" revival recently. Another tincture, Vin Mariana, was made from cocaine and sold as a novelty wine at the end of the nineteenth century. It was quite popular with all classes and endorsed by such notables as Edward Prince of Wales and U.S. President William McKinley.

Social response to alcohol has been variable according to culture and time. It has been totally assimilated into the Mediterranean culture where there exists a low to moderate rate of alcoholism. On the other hand, it is banned in fundamentalist Islamic states. In the United States, it has been identified as a destructive force in the Native American culture. Also in the United States, the Volstead Act of the 1920's was a social experiment to ban the use of alcoholic products. Instead it spawned a unique Prohibition culture based on the alcohol ban itself.

Today, no single alcoholic product is universally banned, although absinthe has near universal prohibition. This light green distillate of wormwood is available only in Portugal and Switzerland. Because of its smell and color, it is often mistaken for chartreuse. Absinthe remains a toxic chemical in spite of its "retro" resurgence in the United States. Chronic use of absinthe produces permanent degenerative changes of the central nervous system. Interestingly, the few remaining bottles of the nineteenth century absinthe "Bois Donc," by the Val Roger distillery in France, are hoarded as collector's items and sold for thousands of dollars.

POPULATIONS AT RISK

Since alcohol is available as a socially accepted beverage, both with meals and at occasions set aside for that purpose (e.g., "wine and cheese parties," "cocktail parties," etc.), it is sometimes difficult to determine demographic data regarding alcohol. Addictive drinking is defined as loss of control manifested by preoccupation with alcohol, compulsive use of alcohol with intoxication, and continuous relapse regarding alcohol use.[4]

Alcohol is the most widely used and abused drug in the Western world. In the United States there is a lifetime prevalence of alcoholism of 13.8 percent. This is distributed between a 23.8 percent prevalence among men but only a 4.6 percent prevalence among women, giving a male to female ratio of 5-to-1. Alcohol abuse begins in youth. By age 19, 40 percent of all abusers have begun to abuse alcohol. By age 30, this reaches 80 percent. After age 60, there is a second, late onset of alcoholism.[5,6,7]

Whereas over one-third of male alcoholics have a co-existing psychiatric disorder, usually sociopathy, 65 percent of female alcoholics have a co-existing psychiatric diagnosis of anxiety and/or depression. Demographically, alcoholism is highest in blue collar males. There is no statistical difference among female alcoholics.[5,8,9]

Based on hospital surveys, it is estimated that 5 to 10 percent of all women drink alcohol to excess during pregnancy. Approximately 3 to 5 percent of these women can be classified as alcoholics. Among 1,000 live births in the United States, as many as three of the children are born with fetal alcohol syndrome. If the aborted fetus were factored in, this percentage would be higher. It is known that among women diagnosed as alcoholics by previous diagnosis or postpartum diagnosis, 5 to 10 percent of them produce babies with fetal alcohol syndrome.[6,10]

Caucasian populations with higher levels of inactive alcohol dehydrogenase-2 tend to have a lower incidence of alcoholism. Low-risk Asian populations also have an atypical aldehyde dehydrogenase as well as relatively high levels of inactive alcohol dehydrogenase.[11]

PHYSIOLOGY

Alcohol acts at two major receptor sites. Like benzodiazepines and the barbiturates, it acts at γ-aminobutyric acid (GABA) receptor channels. In addition, recent research has shown that it also disrupts glutaminergic activity by inhibition of the N-methyl-D-aspartate (NMDA) receptors.[8,11]

Alcohol acts on GABA-receptors, which gate chloride channels, to enhance inhibition. It also inhibits the NMDA receptor to produce supersensitivity of postsynaptic biogenic amine receptors, especially noradrenergic ones. By exciting glutaminergic and GABA-minergic receptors, there is inhibition of dopamine, norepinephrine and serotonin release. Some research has indicated that this action may be mediated solely by glutaminergic action.[3]

Ethanol acts throughout the central nervous system at the site of the GABA-minergic and glutaminergic receptors. Activity sites include the inferior coliculi, mammillary bodies, the hippocampus, septum, locus ceruleus, nucleus accumbens, pars compacta and thalamus.

In addition to activity at receptor sites, alcohol can cause changes in the permeability of the neuronal membrane at both the lipid and protein layers. As a result of this membrane disruption, there is a change in the balance of calcium, potassium and sodium enzymes. This produces inhibition of sodium-activated triphosphatase and potassium-activated triphosphatase. As a result, there is diminished sodium influx and decreased potassium efflux. This, in turn, leads to diminished neuronal impulse conduction and propagation.

Between 90 and 98 percent of ingested alcohol is metabolized by hepatic oxidation at a rate of 1 ml. per 40 minutes. Alcohol is broken down to form acetaldehyde by alcohol dehydrogenase. Acetaldehyde is then broken down to acetate.

Acetaldehyde is a metabolite much more potent than the alcohol itself. It acts to inhibit its own oxidation, it inactivates co-enzyme A, and it interrupts mitochondrial oxidated phosphorylation. With high levels of acetaldehyde, there is increased release of catecholamines and hypoglycemia. At low acetaldehyde levels, catecholamines are preferentially metabolized reductively through oxidation. By reductive metabolism, the catecholamine metabolites react with acetylcholine to produce end-products which may interact with opiate receptors. This may account for opiate cross-reactivity in alcoholism.[11] These products include tetrahydroisoquinoline and salsolinol. This latter compound produces some morphine-like effects and competes with naloxone for μ-opiate receptor sites.

One minor metabolic route is found in the liver and kidneys with peroxisomes and erythrocytes. A second one is in the hepatocytic endoplasmic reticulum. In chronic alcoholism, however, these two systems show increased activity. This is probably an adaptive mechanism to overloading of NADH.

Up to 10 percent of ingested alcohol which is not metabolized is excreted in the urine or in expired air. Expired alcohol is used by law enforcement agencies to determine serum alcohol levels. The amount of alcohol found upon exhalation is multiplied by a factor of 2,300 to calculate the amount of serum alcohol.

In addition to its effects on the brain, alcohol's most well-known effect is the formation of liver cirrhosis. Chronically high levels of acetaldehyde cause an increase in the NADH/NAD ratio, which causes lipogenesis and decreased glycolysis. There are increased levels of all lipids including cholesterol, phospholipids and triglycerides. Over time, hyperlipemia and fatty degeneration results. As the levels of lipids increase, there is an actual deposition of lipid molecules in the liver cells. This produces swelling, displacement and degeneration of the organelles. This fatty infiltration may be associated with hyaline inclusion bodies and a breakdown of the mitochondria in both the smooth and rough endoplasmic reticulum.

Over time, cirrhosis occurs. There is progressive degeneration of the parenchyma accompanied by hypertrophy of the interstitial connective tissue. The liver is initially enlarged and then, as drinking continues, it shrinks into a hard fibrotic mass. This shrinkage produces portal hypertension and development of collateral circulation. In some cases, chronic alcoholism can produce alcoholic hepatitis.

Alcohol also affects the pancreas in like manner causing fibrotic, edematous, atrophic and nephropathic changes. It can also produce cellular infiltration, hemorrhage and necrosis. With alcoholism, 10 percent of patients develop cirrhosis and 10 percent develop chronic pancreatitis, although many cases overlap.

Alcohol is sometimes used to treat heart disease and hyperlipidemia.[12] Alcohol does have a clearing effect upon lipids from the blood stream, and also produces peripheral vasodilatation and diminished vascular resistance.[13] Unfortunately, moderate to high levels of alcohol can alter cardiac cell permeability. This can produce changes in ionization resulting in atrial flutter, fibrillation and/or ventricular tachycardia. If drinking persists, cardiac cell respiration and calcium uptake can be inhibited. In many cases, this is associated with increased levels of intracellular triglycerides producing "alcoholic cardiomyopathy."

MEDICAL COMPLICATIONS

The largest number of complications seen in any drug of abuse occurs with alcohol. Although cirrhosis, pancreatitis and long term central degenerative change are most commonly seen, a number of conditions occur which involve other portions of the gastrointestinal tract, the peripheral nervous system, and the hematopoietic system.

Peripheral Neuropathies

Peripheral neuropathies arise because of deficiencies of various vitamins or minerals. (See also Chapter 19, Nutritional Aspects of Drug Abuse.)

Vitamin B6 (pyridoxine hydrochloride) deficiencies are caused by alcoholic disruption of pyridoxine transamination and decarboxylation. Alcohol also inhibits activation of pyridoxine and pyridoxal phosphate, decreases pyridoxal kinase activity, and increases the rate of metabolism and clearance of pyridoxal phosphate. Acetaldehyde further diminishes pyridoxine levels by displacement of pyridoxal phosphate from binding sites, and by stimulation of pyridoxal phosphate phosphatase. Symptoms seen with diminished pyridoxine levels include parasthesias, numbness, diminished sensation to light touch, and a burning sensation in the soles or the palms.

Folic acid and vitamin B12 (cyanocobalamin) deficiencies produce symptoms similar to that of pyridoxine deficiencies.[14] Generally, deficiencies of these vitamins occur from alcoholic malabsorption and diminished intake. There is also an impaired storage, formation, and release of folic acid and cyanocobalamine, as well as an increased rate of excretion. Interestingly, beer drinkers generally have higher levels of folic acid than other alcoholics because beer itself has a rather high folate content.

Night vision is mediated by retinal. Vitamin A dehydrogenase mediates the transformation of retinol to retinal using zinc as a co-factor. High alcohol intake diminishes vitamin A absorption, activation and storage while it increases metabolism and excretion. It also increases renal clearance of zinc. As a result of deficiencies of this vitamin and this mineral, there is diminution of night vision.

Magnesium is the most common of the alcoholic-induced mineral deficiencies.[15] In addition to the poor nutritional habits of chronic alcoholics, magnesium levels are lowered by malabsorption and increased renal excretion. In some alcoholics, diarrhea may be an additional factor. Irritability and fasciculations are the two most common symptoms. If hypomagnesia occurs in the presence of acidosis, convulsions may ensue. Persistent hypomagnesemia may result in nephrocalcinosis.

Central Nervous System Pathology

Most central pathology seen in alcoholics is caused by vitamin B1 (thiamine) deficiency. Alcoholism is generally associated with decreased absorption and diminished production of thiamine due to thiamine hydrophosphate inhibition. In addition, there may be secondary reduction of thiamine levels due to loss of thiamine storage depots in alcohol-damaged livers.

Wernicke-Korsakoff syndrome is the result of thiamine deficiency. It classically presents as decreased memory (Wernicke syndrome) or memory gaps with confabulation (Korsakoff syndrome). Other symptoms include centrally-mediated ataxia, ophthalmoplegia, nystagmus, ptosis, confusion and stupor.

Major pathological changes occur in the mammillary bodies which may become ischemic, infarcted or thrombotic. In addition, neuronal death and resultant glial infiltration occurs in these bodies as well as in the thalamus, periaqueductal grey matter, vestibular nuclei, cerebellar vermis and the oculomotor nerve nucleus. Lesions of the mammillary bodies and the thalamus produce impairment of memory storage. Ophthalmoplegia and other changes are due to pathology in the oculomotor nerves. Ataxia is due to atrophy of the vermis.[16]

Vitamin B complex (niacin) deficiency, or pellagra, can produce progressive generalized dementia. This degeneration is usually fatal. Other symptoms include diarrhea and dermatitis. A useful mnemonic for pellagra is the 4-D's: diarrhea, dermatitis, dementia and death.

Gastrointestinal Changes

Important gastrointestinal changes take place in the liver, pancreas, esophagus and stomach. The oxidation of alcohol to acetaldehyde causes an increase in the NADH/NAD ratio. This change in the ratio subsequently causes a disruption of the Krebs cycle, producing a shift to the left in the lactate/pyruvate ratio. This shift reduces phagolysis and gluconeogenesis resulting in lipogenesis. As liver cells swell with over-abundant lipid storage, organelles are displaced. With increased damage, hepatitis and cirrhosis can occur. Initially, levels of SGOT and SGPT (serum glutamic oxalacetic transaminase and serum glutamic pyruvic transaminase, respectively), GGT (gammaglutamyl transferase), α-phosphatase and bilirubin are all elevated.[17]

copyright 1997

As the liver continues to fail, the polymorphonuclear leukocyte infiltration accompanies steatosis, necrosis, sclerosis and cholestasis. Histologic studies reveal hyaline inclusion bodies and disruption of mitochondria in the endoplasmic reticula. Continued chemical injury produces scarring usually followed by regeneration. The scarring and the nodular formation occurring during regeneration can produce hypertension in the portal vein as well as in the collateral circulation. These circulatory problems then can produce spider angiomata, caput medusae, telangiectasias and palmar erythema.[18]

Alcohol can disrupt the integrity of the mucosal lining of the gastrointestinal tract, producing irritation, ulceration and bleeding.[19] This process is enhanced by cirrhotic changes. Curling's ulcer, a bleeding of the esophageal varices, is a characteristic finding of chronic alcoholism. Diarrhea can be produced because of the direct effects of the alcohol as well as deficiencies of niacin and magnesium. Vitamin K depletion, which occurs due to the alcoholic-induced death of intestinal flora, can also produce diarrhea and/or steatorrhea. There may also be increased risk of cancer associated with high alcohol use.[20,21]

Although not as common as liver or gastrointestinal pathology, pancreatic injuries are often seen in alcoholics. Generally, alcohol produces spasms of the sphincter of Oddi and an increased release of pancreatic enzymes. The backflow of these enzymes can irritate the pancreas, producing inflammation.

Acute pancreatitis is associated with pancreatic interstitial edema, cellular infiltration, and hemorrhagic changes. Laboratory changes include hypoglycemia, myoglobinuria, proteinuria, and elevated levels of serum and urinary amylase. Pancreatitis is also associated with pulmonary edema, renal failure, pancreatic abscesses, and pseudocysts. Acute pancreatitis presents with severe abdominal pain most notable in the back, accompanied by diaphoresis, fever, nausea, and vomiting. It is sometimes mistaken for acute appendicitis since it is associated with rebound tenderness, guarding and diminished bowel sounds.

Chronic relapsing pancreatitis is associated with obstructions of the pancreatic duct. As a result, there is increased cellular infiltration and metaplasia of the pancreas with progressive necrosis, fibrosis and edema of the pancreas as well as dilatation of the pancreatic ducts. The clinical picture is similar to that of acute pancreatitis except for malabsorption of fat and protein, producing steatorrhea.

Cardiovascular Changes

Changes in the cardiovascular system can be produced by direct or indirect effects of alcohol. Oxidation of alcohol produces acetaldehyde and acetate, which can increase cardiac output and cause vasodilation. These effects are in contrast to the direct depressive effects of alcohol on myocardial tissue. Acetaldehyde may also alter the sinoatrial node, producing atrial fibrillation, atrial flutter and, by actions throughout the conduction bundles and nodes, ventricular tachycardia. Alcoholic-induced hypomagnesemia can also produce arrhythmias.[22]

Alcoholic cardiomyopathy is generally found in patients who have chronically high levels of alcohol intake. Alcohol intake at this level produces inhibition of both myocardial cell respiration and calcium intake. In addition, there is triglyceride accumulation. Auscultation reveals diminished S1, systolic murmur, and gallop of S3 and S4. There is also lateral displacement of the apical pulse and diminished force of the carotid pulse. An EKG generally records atrial ventricular arrhythmias, conduction delays, and diminished voltage.

Over time, as the drinking history progresses, there is a symmetrical enlargement of the heart. In the end stage, there is right-sided heart failure, pulmonary hypertension, and chronic ischemia. Death usually occurs from ventricular arrhythmias.[12,23] As discussed in the gastrointestinal subsection, portal hypertension is the result of cirrhotic nodular formation.[24]

Dermatological Changes

Many of the changes seen in the skin are a result of hepatic effects. These include palmar arrhythmia, spider angiomata, telangiectasias and caput medusae. Other liver changes involve hyperplasia of the palmar fascia, producing Dupuytren's contracture.

Generalized dermatitis is also seen with niacin, zinc and vitamin A deficiencies. In addition, vitamin A deficiency is associated with skin dryness and hyperkeratosis. A deficiency of vitamin C can produce similarly dry skin and hyperkeratosis as well as subperiosteal and gingival bleeding. Poor wound healing is associated with both vitamin C and zinc deficiency.

Musculoskeletal Changes

Most visible changes seen in the muscular system are produced by magnesium deficiency. Magnesium can produce irritability of all muscles including the heart, fasiculations and, rarely, formications. Due to the presence of formications and fasiculations, alcoholic hypomagnesemia is sometimes confused with cocaine withdrawal. Direct alcoholic changes upon enzymes may produce peripheral myopathies with resultant inflammation. Inflammatory changes and necrosis can, in turn, produce persisting tenderness. In the laboratory, chronic muscle tissue damage can be diagnosed by elevations of CPK levels and, later, myoglobinuria. An often-overlooked result of myopathy is the disruption of uterine contractions.

Hematopoietic Changes

Alcohol acts both directly and indirectly upon bone marrow and lymphatic tissue to cause changes in the production of red blood cells, white blood cells, and platelets. In addition, there are changes in blood clotting which are not directly dependent upon platelet functioning.

Red blood cell changes can include both macrocytic and microcytic anemia. Microcytic anemia is not usually due to iron depletion. In fact, many alcoholic beverages, especially red wines, are themselves sources of iron. In addition, serum iron levels may be increased as a function of increased absorption due to folic acid deficiency, pancreatic disease, liver disease and increased secretion of gastric acid. Generally, when iron deficiency does occur, it is usually due to gastrointestinal bleeding. Usually alcoholic microcytosis is caused by inhibition of heme synthesis.

Deficiencies of vitamin B12 and folic acid can produce macrocytosis or macrocytic anemia. Normocytic and microcytic anemia may also result from a direct alcoholic effect on hematopoiesis, causing erythrocyte fragility and erythrocyte sequestration in the spleen.

Suppression of bone marrow functioning can also reduce the formation and functioning of leukocytes, macrophages (killer cells) and lymphocytes. Granulocytic migration to sites of infection or injury is slowed, and immune status may be compromised.[25]

Alcohol may produce abnormalities in vitamin K-dependent coagulation factors VII, IX, and X. Direct action of alcohol can decrease the rate of platelet production and produce thrombocytopenia. As a result of changes in coagulation factors and platelets, prothrombin time may be prolonged.

Endocrine Effects

Most of the alcohol-induced endocrine effects are seen in the steroidal hormones, i.e., those of the adrenals, ovaries and testicles.[26] Disruption of normal hypothalamic-pituitary-target organ function reduces the level of testosterone in men, and follicle-stimulating hormone and luteinizing hormone in women.

In men with cirrhosis, precursors of testosterone and other male hormones are shunted to estrogen formation. This produces demasculinization with subsequent gynecomastia, muscle wasting and redistribution of male fat- and hair-patterns. Hepatic synthesis of testosterone is also reduced and inactivated by decrements in liver functioning. Alcohol can also directly cause injury to the seminiferous tubules, Leydig's cells, and the germinal epithelia, thus producing decreased testosterone and diminished sperm count.

Axial changes in women can produce decreased lubrication, impairment of vaginal pressure, decreased orgasmic receptivity and diminished libido. There is temporary or permanent infertility and menstrual dysfunction. Alcohol also stimulates the hypothalamic-pituitary-adrenal axis to produce ACTH and cortisol. In chronic alcoholism, this can give a Cushing-like syndrome.

Oxidation of alcohol shifts corticosteroid metabolic pathways to the reductive rather than the oxidative modes. This can be measured by increased production of one catecholamine metabolite, MHPG, and decreased production of a second, VMA. Because of these reductive changes, there are increased insulin levels, increased glycogen break-down in the liver and resultant hypoglycemia. Because of this, many chronically malnourished alcoholics present with ketonic dehydration.

Withdrawal/Delirium Tremens

Alcoholic withdrawal, especially in its most extreme form, delirium tremens (DT's), can be life threatening. Alcohol acts indirectly on chloride channels through glutamic and GABA-minergic receptor cites. As alcohol assumes regulatory functions over chloride channels, endogenous production of GABA and glutamate is reduced. When alcohol is suddenly withdrawn, chloride suppression of activating neurotransmitters such as indolamines and catecholamines ceases. This then produces the withdrawal process.

With withdrawal, central control of coordination and temperature homeostasis is suddenly disrupted. This produces the characteristic presentation of tremors, diaphoresis, and hyperpyrexia. Delirium tremens is the production of a delirious state associated with tremors and is the most severe form of alcohol withdrawal. Seizures may occur in severe alcoholic withdrawal and are occasionally fatal if not treated.[27,28]

MEDICAL MANAGEMENT

Management of the alcoholic involves the treatment of withdrawal and replenishment of nutritional deficiencies. A variety of substances can be used to detoxify the withdrawing patient.

For traditional reasons as well as ease of management, benzodiazepines are generally employed. Historically, Librium (chlordiazepoxide) is most often used. Chlordiazepoxide 10 mg. to 100 mg. three times a day to every four hours (not to exceed 300 mg. per day) is prescribed on a mandated or as-needed titration-downward basis. Generally, detoxification can be accomplished within three to seven days.

Breakthrough seizures, hyperpyrexia (greater than 101°F), and hallucinations are managed by as-needed administration of chlordiazepoxide. If there is a risk of seizures, the physician should order seizure precautions according to institutional protocols. If break-through seizures, hyperpyrexia or hallucinations should occur, as-needed doses of chlordiazepoxide should be applied at a dosage equal to one mandated dose.

Many clinicians prefer to use lorazepam. Lorazepam has the advantage of being the only commonly available benzodiazepine that may be administered on an intramuscular basis without complication if acute administration is necessary. The dosage ranges from .5 to 2 mg. three times a day to every six hours (not to exceed 10 mg. per day).

Although all benzodiazepines may be administered intravenously, inexperienced personnel may produce respiratory arrest by accelerated push. Benzodiazepines generally work upon GABA-minergic sites to re-regulate the chloride channels. Similar effects can be produced by paraldehyde and chloral hydrate. Paraldehyde, because of light and temperature sensitivity, is not to be recommended for detoxification under any circumstances. Chloral hydrate can be administered orally, rectally, intramuscularly or intravenously at dosages ranging from 250 mg. to 650 mg.

Other novel medications may be used for detoxification. The beta-blockers, atenolol and propranolol, are useful. These medications block the β-adrenergic receptor sites to reduce the rate and amount of catecholamine release.

Clonidine, an antihypertensive agent and an α-adrenergic agonist, operates at the locus ceruleus to down-regulate production and release of catecholamines. The dosage is 17 μg. per kg. in four divided dosages. Downward titration usually takes place over a five-day period.

The antiepileptic compound, carbamazepine, operates by reducing kindling[4] and is prescribed at an initial dosage of 100 mg. to 300 mg. every six to eight hours, not to exceed 1200 mg. a day. Depakene or valproic acid operates by similar mechanisms and at similar dosage levels.

In areas of central Europe where benzodiazepines have been in short supply, intravenous use of magnesium sulfate has been employed with great success. Magnesium can either be treated by infusion or by intravenous injection of magnesium sulfate at the rate of 1 to 4 or more grams of the salt per day. Magnesium operates by reducing the release of catecholamines, indolamines, and acetylcholine at neuronal and neuromuscular junctions. It reduces tremors and is an excellent anticonvulsant.[12]

Occasionally, metronidazole is dissolved in alcoholic beverages. This produces a potent cocktail sometimes called a "PJ." Its effects include flushing, disorientation, excitation, tachycardia and elevated blood pressure. It does not require special intervention.[29]

The most common nutritional deficiencies are thiamine, folic acid, and magnesium. Thiamine deficiencies can be treated by thiamine 200 mg. intramuscularly for three days followed by 200 mg. orally for six months to five years. Folate and vitamin B12 deficiencies can be treated by vitamin B12 1 to 2 cc intramuscularly followed by folic acid 1 mg. every day for six months to a year. Hypomagnesemia is treated by magnesium sulfate injection 1000 mg. intramuscularly in alternating buttocks over a two- to five-day period. Maintenance can be accomplished by prescription of magnesium oxide 250 mg. every day.

Niacin deficiency or pellagra is generally treated by oral application of inositol hexaniacinate at a daily dosage range of 200 mg. to 300 mg. Pyridoxine (vitamin B6) is treated orally at a dosage range of 25 mg. every day. Vitamin C deficiencies are treated with 35 mg. every day. Zinc deficiencies are treated orally with 15 mg. every day.

Anemia and changes in erythrocyte morphology can complicate management of patients with sickle cell and Von Gierke's disease, precipitating an acute crisis. In all cases of vitamin or mineral deficiency, the physician should work with the dietitian to develop a specific diet which can alleviate these deficiencies (see Chapter 19). These deficiencies may also be compounded by a concurrent eating disorder (see Chapter 15).

TYPICAL CASE PRESENTATION

The patient was a 31-year-old white male who presented to the emergency room complaining of visual hallucinations of "animals all over the road running in front of my car." He was agitated and mildly aggressive. Heart rate and blood pressure were mildly elevated but axillary temperature was 100.5°F. As a result of his presentation, he was triaged to the psychiatric service.

The psychiatry resident noted that speech was pressured, content mildly delusional with visual though not auditory hallucinations. History was negative for previous psychiatric disorder, alcohol abuse or drug abuse. A SMAC-23, CBC-Diff and urine drug and alcohol screen were then ordered on a stat basis and the patient was placed in a holding area.

The drug screen was negative but the CBC-Diff demonstrated macrocytic anemia. The SMAC had numerous abnormal findings, including elevated liver function tests (LFT), elevated gamma-glutamyltransferase levels (GGT), and decreased magnesium levels. On the basis of these findings, the patient was determined to be in early alcohol withdrawal.

The resident then presented the patient with the findings and presumptive diagnosis. Confronted with these results, the patient admitted to an eleven-year history of alcohol abuse. He had increased his intake to one-and-a-half pints of vodka per day for the past year. Due to marital pressures, he had attempted to detoxify himself. This was attempted without medical supervision due to fear of discovery of his alcoholism by his employer.

After lengthy discussion, the patient agreed to be voluntarily admitted to the hospital addiction recovery unit. After a 30 minute bureaucratic delay, he was transferred. On admission to the unit, vital signs were taken. It was noted that at this time axillary temperatures had increased to 101.5°F and coarse resting tremors were present. The patient continued to have coarse resting tremors. It was now determined that his alcohol withdrawal had advanced to delirium tremens. He was noticeably diaphoretic and complained of being light-headed.

He was given an immediate injection of lorazepam 2 mg. intramuscularly. He was then transported immediately to a bed on the unit. Here he was placed on seizure precautions. Chlordiazepoxide 50 mg. orally every 6 hours was ordered with vital signs every 4 hours. In the event that the body temperature exceeded 101°F or the patient manifested coarse tremors, convulsions, or visual hallucinations, an additional 50 mg. of chlordiazepoxide was to be given and the house officer called. The chlordiazepoxide was then ordered to be titrated downward at 20 percent of the previous dosage each day unless withdrawal symptoms developed.

An additional history and complete physical examination were done. In addition to the previous medical history, he complained of "blackouts" with occasional confabulation. He had numbness in his legs and feet. A physical examination revealed horizontal nystagmus, fasciculations over the deltoids and left pectoralis major, bilateral calf tenderness and absent vibratory sensation in both legs.

Macrocytic anemia was treated with 1 mg. of vitamin B12 intramuscularly on an acute basis. This was followed by folic acid 1 mg. every day, by mouth. The amnestic episodes complicated by confabulation (Wernicke-Korsakoff syndrome) were treated with thiamine 200 mg. intramuscularly for three days followed by thiamine 200 mg. every day orally thereafter. The hypomagnesemia was next treated by magnesium sulfate 1000 mg. intramuscularly every day in alternating buttocks over a five-day period.

The dietitian next assessed the patient. He recommended a diet high in magnesium sources including nuts, freeze dried coffee and dark vegetables such as kale.

During his hospitalization, he participated in group and individual therapy sessions trying to understand his helplessness. He had a history of multiple discontinuances despite marital, vocational and sexual difficulties. He finally accepted that his use of alcohol was a cause and not a result of those difficulties. After his acceptance of personal responsibility, his wife agreed to enter family-group therapy. While still an inpatient, the patient began attending in-hospital Alcoholics Anonymous meetings and his wife attended Al-Anon meetings. After 14 days, he was discharged with nutritional supplements and dietary suggestions. He was referred to his family physician for monitoring of thiamine, vitamin B12/folic acid and magnesium levels. He agreed to continue attendance at AA meetings.

NOTES

1. Buck F. Bring 'Em Back Alive! NY: MacMillan, 1935.
2. Gullberg RG. Duplicate breath alcohol analysis: some further parameters for evaluation. Med Sci Law 1991; **31(3)**: 226-8.
3. AJ Giannini, AE Slaby, MC Giannini. Overdose and Detoxification Emergencies. New Hyde Park: Medical Examination, 1982.
4. Alcohol problems in the general hospital. Drug Ther Bull 1991; **29(18)**: 69-71.
5. Glass TA, Prigerson H, Kasl SV, Mendes de Leon CF. The effects of negative life events on alcohol consumption among older men and women. J Gerontol 1995; **50(4)**: S205-16.
6. Donnermeyer JF, Park DS. Alcohol use among rural adolescents; predictive and situational factors. Int J Addict 1995; **30(4)**: 459-79.
7. Flannery MT, Altus P,Taub LD. Alcohol withdrawal with an unusual presentation. South Med J 1991; **84(11)**: 1408-9.
8. Wechsler H, Dowdall GW, Davenport A, Rimm EB. A gender-specific measure of binge drinking among college students. Am J Public Health 1995; **85(7)**: 982-5.
9. Escobedo LG, Chorba TL, Wasweller R. Patterns of alcohol use and the risk of drinking and driving among US high school students. Am J Publ Health 1995; **85(7)**: 976-8.
10. Duffy JC. Alcohol consumption and all-cause mortality. Int J Epidemiol 1995; **24(1)**: 100-5.
11. Tsai G, Gastfriend D, Coyle J. The glutaminergic basis of human alcoholism. Am J Psychiatry, 1995; **152(3)**: 332-40.
12. Stockwell TR, Lang E, Lewis PN. Is wine the drink of moderation? Med J Aust 1995; **162(11)**: 578, 580-581.

13. Ridker PM, Vaughan DE, Stampfer MJ, Glynn RJ, Hennekens CH. Association of moderate alcohol consumption and plasma concentration of endogenous tissue-type plasminogen activator. JAMA 1994; **272(12)**: 929-33.

14. Wu AH, Henderson BE. Alcohol and tobacco use: risk factors for colorectal adenoma and carcinoma? J Natl Cancer Inst 1995; **87(4)**: 239-40.

15. Fink EB. Mineral metabolism in alcoholism. In: Kissin B, Begleiter H (Eds.), The Biology of Alcoholism. NY: Plenum Press, 1971. Pp. 377-389.

16. Rindi G, Ventura U. Thiamine intestinal transport. Physiol Rev 1972; **52**: 821-827.

17. Dimanowski UA, Stickel F, Maier H. Gärtner U, Seitz HK. Effect of alcohol on gastrointestinal cell regeneration as a possible mechanism in alcohol-associated carcinogenesis. Alcohol 1995; **12(2)**: 111-115.

18. Lieber CS. Hepatic, metabolic and toxic effects of ethanol: 1991 Update. Alcohol Clin Exp Res 1991; **15(4)**: 573-92.

19. Eastwood GL. Epithelial renewal in protection and repair of gastroduodenal mucosa. J Clin Gastroenterol 1991; **1**: S48-53.

20. Lin HJ, Lee FY, Lee CH, Lee SD. Endoscopic injection of alcohol to stop peptic ulcer hemorrhage. J Clin Gastroenterol 1991; **13(4)**: 376-9.

21. Seulrud M, Mendoza S, Rossiter G, Gelrud D. Rossiter A, Souney PF. Effect of local instillation of alcohol on sphincter of Oddi motor activity: combined ERCP and manometry study. Gastrointest Endosc 1991; **37(4)**: 428-32.

22. Brugada P. Alcohol ablation of atrioventricular conduction. Br Heart J 1991; **66(3)**: 257-8.

23. Bertolet BD, Freund G, Martin CA, Perchalski, DL, Williams CM, Pepine CJ. Unrecognized left ventricular dysfunction in an apparently health alcohol abuse population. Drug Alcohol Depend 1991; **28(2)**: 113-119.

24. Kochhar R, Goenka MK, Mehta SK. Outcome of injection sclerotherapy using absolute alcohol in patients with cirrhosis, non-cirrhotic portal fibrosis, and extrahepatic portal venous obstruction. Gastrointest Endosc 1991; **37(4)**: 460-4.

25. Stibler H; Beaugè F, Leguicher A, Borg S. Biophysical and biochemical alterations in erythrocyte membranes from chronic alcoholics. Scand J Clin Lab Invest 1991; **51(4)**: 309-19.

26. Lichtigfield FJ, Gillman MA. Advances in understanding alcohol withdrawal states. Postgrad Med J 1991; **67**: 700-1.

27. Fujiwar T, Watanabe M, Matsude K, Senbongi M, Yagi K, Seino M. Complex partial status epilepticus provoked by ingestion of alcohol: a case report. Epilepsia 1991; **32(5)**: 650-6.

28. Nuñez-Vergara LJ, Yudelevich J, Squella JA, Speisky H. Drug-acetaldehyde interactions during ethanol metabolism *in vitro*. Alcohol 1991; **(2)**: 139-46.

29. Giannini AJ, DeFrance DT. Metronidazole and alcohol: potential for combinative abuse. J Toxicol: Clin Toxicol 1984; **20**: 509-515.

CHAPTER 3

AMPHETAMINES

Amphetamine belongs to a group of recreational drugs called the sympathomimetics. The sympathomimetic cocaine is discussed in Chapter 6, and the sympathomimetic khat, in Chapter 7.

Most of the drugs of abuse discussed in this book either minimize or distort reality. In contradistinction, amphetamine and the other sympathomimetics intensify it. They give the abuser increased physical and mental energy. There is an intensification of libido and aggressivity. Fatigue and hunger are temporarily minimized.

Amphetamine is used for a variety of purposes. Some abusers use it to increase *joie de vivre*. By minimizing the need for sleep, rest and food, it can maximize endurance. In street parlance, the amphetamine user is "wired." These wiring effects are truly electrifying.

Amphetamine is at times seen as an occupational requirement. Truck drivers utilize amphetamine to squeeze extra miles out of long distance hauls; students utilize it to ward off the need for sleep when pulling all-nighters during finals week; and medical interns utilize it to get through 72 hours of weekend call.

Amphetamine brings the abuser "up." But the laws of physics decree that eventually the abuser must come down or "crash." With the depletion of catecholamines, the abuser must either increase the dosage or go through a period of profound lethargy. Irritability induced by chronic amphetamine abuse led to the late sixties' aphorism, "speed kills."

how quaint

LABORATORY TESTING[1,2]

In testing for amphetamine, urine samples are preferred to serum samples because of concentration of this compound during renal clearance. For qualitative analysis, thin-layer chromatography (TLC) can be utilized to provide a quick and inexpensive method of detection. Quantitative analysis may be performed by radioimmunoassay (RIA) or the enzyme multiple immunoassay test (EMIT). Unlike TLC, both EMIT and RIA can be used with either serum or urine samples and do not require prior extraction.

EMIT has a sensitivity level of 2 μg. per ml. while RIA has a sensitivity of 1 μg. per ml. Although these methods may be used to analyze serum samples, their relatively poor sensitivity renders then unsuitable. In addition, these two immunoassay techniques have a high degree of cross-sensitivity. A number of substances allowable in the workplace such as phenylpropanolamine, pseudoephedrine, cinnamedryl and phenylephrine cross react in the EMIT and RIA to produce false positives.

Gas liquid chromatography (GLC) tends to be more specific and more sensitive but is rather expensive and requires prior extraction. When a high degree of sensitivity is needed, a combination of gas/liquid chromatography combined with mass spectrometry (GLC/MS) provide the techniques of choice. Generally, this latter method is used only to confirm results of other techniques. Its main utility is in the legal spheres.

HISTORY

The first description of an amphetamine-like compound was in the *Herbal*, written by the Chinese emperor Nung in 2737 B.C. In 1887, I. Edeleanu synthesized amphetamine. Fifty-six years later, G.A. Alles published a paper on the actions of the sympathomimetic phenylisopropanolamine. Two years later M. Prinzmetal described the use of benzedrine in the treatment of narcolepsy.[3]

Also during the nineteen-forties, G. Piness reviewed an 1895 publication of George Oliver and Edward A. Schaefer which described the actions and interrelationship of the adrenal corticotropic hormones upon the central nervous system. In his review, he was able to relate actions of sympathomimetics to those of the adrenal corticotropic hormones. Soon afterwards, benzedrine and amphetamine entered the pharmacopeia of recreational drugs.[3]

In the 1930's, the major attraction of amphetamine was its stimulant effect. Amphetamine was initially seen as a middle- and upper-class drug. An analogue of amphetamine called benzedrine was sniffed in inhalers specifically designed for this purpose. Indeed, benzedrine inhalers became popular and leading jewelers in New York, London, Paris and Florence manufactured silver, gold and platinum devices for the fashionable benzedrine addict. Many contemporaries wrote of the use of benzedrine inhalers by gamblers at the gaming tables of Monte Carlo.[4]

Amphetamine was also used during World War II by elite German soldiers. It is assumed that in the latter days of the Third Reich, Adolph Hitler abused amphetamine to deal with the mounting pressures of Germany's implosion.[5]

In the post-war period, amphetamine became a chemical crutch utilized by long distance truck drivers to try to meet impossible deadlines. Its use was chronicled in such truck driving songs as *Six Days on the Road* by Waylon Jennings. In the sixties, amphetamine became part of the psychedelic subculture of the hippie movement. It was used for its stimulant effects as well as its ability to prolong the effects of hallucinogenic compounds.

In the fifties and sixties, amphetamine was legally prescribed and subsequently abused by obese patients. It was overprescribed by naive physicians and not-quite naive diet doctors.

Amphetamine has been manufactured in either racemic or dextro-form. The racemic mixture is benzedrine. The dextro-form is sold under the trade name Dexedrine and was vended for its anorectic effect. Methedrine is a methylated amphetamine derivative sold because of its central effect. Methoxylation of amphetamine produces MDA (methylene dioxy amphetamine) which is discussed in Chapter 11, Psychedelics. Methamphetamine and methoxylated amphetamine became popular in the sixties.

DEMOGRAPHICS[6-8]

Amphetamine use grew in the United States until the mid-sixties when amphetamines were classified as a Schedule II drug. Since then, recreational drug users have taken different paths to obtain amphetamine or amphetamine-like effects. Some have used high doses of over-the-counter analogues such as phenylpropanolamine (PPA) or cinnamedryl. Phenylpropanolamine is used as an anorectic and as a common-cold preparation. Cinnamedryl is used for menstrual cramping. PPA is abused throughout the U.S. Cinnamedryl is abused chiefly in the Southeastern United States, both for anorectic and stimulant effects.[9]

These drugs are obtained in a number of ways. Addicts can get legalized prescriptions of Schedule II drugs from naive or unscrupulous doctors; steal the drugs from hospital formularies; smuggle the drugs into the United States from other countries; or manufacture the drugs in illicit laboratories. Unlike cocaine and phencyclidine, no unified distribution system has evolved. Amphetamine may be manufactured and distributed by cocaine dealers, gangs and other organized crime (see Table 3-1).

Approximately 10 percent of the United States population has abused amphetamine by the age of 30. This high percentage is distorted by high-risk populations. Students, long-distance truck drivers and athletes competing in endurance sports tend to use amphetamine on a chronic or subchronic basis.

Amphetamine is also used in combination with sedative-hypnotics, benzodiazepines or alcohol. Generally, the amphetamine is used to start the day and one of the other, more sedating drugs is used to come down at night. The group utilizing amphetamines in this manner tends to include men whose vocation requires long hours, maximum alertness and minimum fatigue. A smaller group that chronically abuses amphetamine for its anorectic effect is generally white, female and college-educated.

Table 3-1: Proprietary Amphetamine and Other Sympathomimetics Available in the U.S.

Brand Name	Generic Name	Route of Administration
Addenal	Methamphetamine	oral
Atrophil	Phenylpropanolamine	oral
Benzedrine*	Amphetamine	oral
Biphetamine	Dextroamphetamine	oral
Cylert	Pemoline	oral
Desoxyn	Methamphetamine	oral
Dexedrine	Dextroamphetamine	oral
Dextrim	Phenylpropanolamine	oral
Dextrostat	Dextroamphetamine	oral
Entex	Phenylephrine, phenylpropanolamine	oral
Fetamin	Methamphetamine	oral
Midol	Cinnamedryl	oral
Ornade	Phenylpropanolamine	oral
Ritalin	Methylphenidate	oral
Triaminic	Phenylpropanolamine	oral
Vanex Forte	Phenylpropanolamine	oral

*Available only through illicit sources.

PHARMACOLOGY

The pharmacology of amphetamine is similar to that of cocaine in the production of intoxication, tolerance and addiction (see Chapter 6, Cocaine).[10] Approximately 30 percent of amphetamine is absorbed orally and intravenously it is completely absorbed. In both cases, bodywide distribution occurs. Both central and peripheral effects are directly proportional to serum concentration. After amphetamine is ingested, peak concentration levels are reached within 75 or 80 minutes. Protein binding is approximately 20 percent. Intravenous injection is directly absorbed but intramuscular injection is dependent upon muscle perfusion. After intravenous injection, peak levels are achieved in only 30 minutes. The elimination half-life is approximately 4 hours in chronic abusers and 3.5 to 3.8 hours in occasional or naive abusers. Amphetamine is an alkaline molecule (pKa 9.5) much more basic than phencyclidine. The urine pH thus determines ionization and clearance. In acidic urine, the ionized amphetamine molecules are readily excreted. In alkaline urine, non-ionized molecules are reabsorbed by the renal tubules.[11]

The major metabolic pathways of amphetamine and its analogues are the oxidation of the N-atom, and deamination and dealkalization of the α-C. Minor routes of metabolism include N-dealkalization, aromatic hydroxylation, N-oxidation and N-conjugation.

There is no major school of thought regarding the unique concept of "reverse tolerance" in amphetamine. Some researchers have reported that chronic administration of amphetamine produces an increased half-life for amphetamine with a corresponding increase in the amount of nonmetabolized amphetamine that is excreted. However, the bulk of research indicates that the phenomenon of tolerance applies in the same manner for amphetamine as in all addicting situations. Neurotransmitter studies reveal dopaminergic depletion at presynaptic sites as well as postsynaptic supersensitivity.

MEDICAL COMPLICATIONS

See the section, "Medical Complications," in Chapter 7, Cocaine.

DIAGNOSIS

Amphetamine use produces quite different presentations depending upon whether it is an acute, chronic or withdrawal state. Acute single-dosing of amphetamine produces a manic-like state. The patient displays increased activity, poor judgement, impulsivity especially of a sexual nature, lability, pressured speech, loquaciousness, and euphoria. In naive users, there may be anxiety, confusion, suspiciousness and occasionally frank paranoia.

Examination usually reveals increased deep tendon reflexes, hypertonicity, mydriasis, and resting tremors. The skin is generally cool and not flushed. Both diastolic and systolic blood pressure is raised. Heart rate is generally increased. Laboratory testing reveals increased cortisol levels and consequently increased glucose levels. This is a direct sympathomimetic response. Generally, EKG's show paroxysmal atrial tachycardia and premature ventricular contraction.[12]

The chronic abuser, on the other hand, generally presents with a history of constipation and urinary retention. The spouse or lover may describe jerking movements during sleep as well as nocturnal bruxism. Long-term chronic use is also associated with nausea, emesis and, at times, vertigo. Headaches may be of a band-constricting nature, dull or occasionally sharp pain anywhere within the nuchal-cranial area. There is generalized anorexia with possible malnutrition.

Although some patients remain in a panicky state, most are generally depressed. Occasionally, auditory and visual hallucinations are seen. Grand mal seizures may also be reported.

Physical examination of chronic abusers reveals a body temperature in excess of 99 degrees, rapid heart rate, rapid breathing and dilation of the pupils. The patient tends to be hyperalert. Gait is generally ataxic and Romberg's sign is invariably present. There may be stereotypy and/or random jerking movements or bruxism. Nonspecific dermatitis may be present in generalized or localized distribution. There is flushing and the skin feels generally warm. Blood pressure is usually reduced. Tachycardia with PAC's, PVC's and ectopy may be seen on the EKG.

Withdrawal symptoms tend to mimic those of chronic abuse. Also there may be production of formications and phenomena similar to "cocaine bugs" where small, darting objects are seen. There is overeating associated with a craving for sweet, salty or oily foods. The patient in withdrawal has a curious admixture of manic and depressive symptoms. Frank resting, intention and physiological tremors are present. Occasionally, the depressive state may approach suicidal proportions.

TREATMENT

Treatment of acute amphetamine intoxication is somewhat different than that of the other popular sympathomimetics, cocaine and khat. Cocaine is generally too expensive, even in crack form, to produce hypotensive responses. The low concentration availability of cathinone in khat generally makes the amount of leaves necessary to produce severe physical effects beyond the abilities of the human mandible.

Amphetamine overdose, however, is both financially and physiologically accessible. If the patient acutely ingests large amounts of amphetamine, emesis may be induced with syrup of ipecac. If the patient is comatose or convulsing because of acute ingestion, intubation is mandatory. Activated charcoal followed by gastric lavage should eliminate a large fraction of the ingested amphetamine. Although a large number of cathartics may be employed, magnesium sulfate 30 grams is the standard treatment.

If hypotension is present, administer saline and titrate against blood pressure. Generally, this will be sufficient. If the patient does not respond to saline, however, add phentolamine, an alpha-adrenergic blocker, and titrate against blood pressure. If the patient has symptoms of atonic bladder, utilize the saline line and inject with furosemide.

To enhance excretion of amphetamine and its metabolites, produce ion trapping by acidification. Ascorbic acid intramuscularly initially followed by another dose every 12 hours should be sufficient. Some authors advise ammonium chloride, but ascorbic acid is generally safer and does not cause the occasional complication of metabolic acidosis.

The bromocriptine/desipramine protocol can be used for amphetamine detoxification. Since amphetamine produces dopamine depletion, the dopamine agonist, bromocriptine, can quantitatively and qualitatively block the majority of withdrawal symptoms. Desipramine, a noradrenergic agonist, can reduce amphetamine cravings by producing β-adrenergic and dopaminergic receptor subsensitivity.

Table 3-2: Recommended Bromocriptine-Desipramine Protocol for Amphetamine Detox

Day	Bromocriptine Dosage	Desipramine Dosage
1	2.5 mg. four times daily	50 mg. at bedtime
2	1.25 mg. four times daily	50 mg. at bedtime
3	1.25 mg. four times daily	100 mg. at bedtime
4	.625 mg. four times daily	100 mg. at bedtime
5	.625 mg. three times daily	150 mg. at bedtime
6	.625 mg. twice daily	200 mg. at bedtime
7	.625 mg. per day	200 mg. at bedtime
8	Discontinue	Continue for 1 to 8 mos.

The suggested bromocriptine-desipramine protocol for amphetamine is presented in Table 3-2. While the patient is detoxified, nutritional support should be provided. Unless the patient is diabetic, there is no reason to restrict caloric intake. Specific cravings such as those previously mentioned for sweet, salty or other foods, should be satisfied since they probably represent a corrective response to specific deficiencies. If complications such as hypertension and atonic bladder occur, detoxification is generally accomplished on an inpatient unit. As with other drugs, a team approach should be employed.

TYPICAL CASE PRESENTATION

The patient was a 34-year-old black female who was brought to the emergency room. According to her secretary, she had been presiding over a staff meeting when she remarked, "Oh, I'm dizzy" and then passed out.

Examination revealed a thin woman. She was conscious but disoriented to place and situation. Vital signs showed a heart rate of 94, blood pressure of 90 over 40, respirations of 30 per minute, and temperature of 100.4°F. Skin was dry, warm and flushed with a rash over the shoulders and breasts and in the axillary areas. Her pupils were dilated, sclera were non-icteric. Heart rate was rapid but otherwise unremarkable.

An intravenous line of 0.9 saline was inserted and run at 150 cc/hr. An SMAC, CBC-Diff, and U/A were ordered. Urine and serum drug screens were drawn for stat TLC analysis. Within 20 minutes, the patient was conscious though not fully alert. She denied any history of seizures, hypotension, hypoglycemia, diabetes or drug abuse. Shortly thereafter, the results of initial testing revealed low blood sugar, low albumin, low globulin, normocytic anemia and decreased chloride. Drug screens were not available. Her blood pressure at this time was 105 over 65, and the pulse was 85 beats per minute. Respirations were 25 per minute and her temperature remained at 100.4°F.

The patient at this time revealed that she had been dieting because of a new relationship. She denied using diet pills. It was noted at this time that her speech was pressured and that she gestured with an odd jerky movement. A brief neurological examination revealed hyperreflexia but no clonus or Babinski reflex. While the neurological examination was being conducted, the urine and serum drug screens were completed and found to be positive for amphetamine.

The patient then admitted that she had been taking diet pills from two doctors she knew and buying Ritalin from her sister's roommate. In an effort to control her appetite, she discovered that these medications increased her energy level and decreased her need for sleep. After discussing the situation with her parents by telephone, she admitted to a 28-month addiction and agreed to inpatient detoxification.

She was initially detoxified with bromocriptine 2.5 mg. every eight hours orally. During withdrawal, she began experiencing intense hunger which caused great psychological distress because of the patient's fear of getting fat. She also noted formication and emerging dysphoria which was most intense in the evening. The bromocriptine was adjusted downward over a period of 10 days.

Because of the emerging dysphoria, desipramine therapy was instituted. The initial dosage was 50 mg. before bedtime, and this was gradually raised to 200 mg. before bedtime. A psychiatrist was consulted to help the patient deal with her self-image.

The patient refused inpatient or outpatient drug rehabilitation. She did however agree to follow-up therapy with the psychiatrist who had treated her during detoxification.

NOTES

1. Smith FP, Kidwell DA. Isomeric amphetamines — a problem for urinalysis? Forensic Sci Int 1991; **50(2)**: 153-65.
2. Hughes R, Hughes A, Levine B, Smith ML. Stability of phencyclidine and amphetamines in urine specimens. Clin Chem 1991; **37(12)**: 2141-2.
3. Blashko H, Muscholl E. Handbuch Experimental Pharmakalogy. Berlin: Springer-Verlag, 1972.
4. Galbraith JK. A Life in Our Times. Boston: Houghton Mifflin, 1981.
5. Strong K. Intelligence at the Top: The Recollections of a British Intelligence Officer. Garden City, NY: Doubleday, 1960.
6. Bell P. The precipitants of amphetamine addiction. Brit J Psychiatry 1971; **119**: 171-180.
7. Wright JD, Pearl L. Knowledge and experience of young people regarding drug abuse, 1969-89. BMJ 1991; **300(67)**: 99-103.
8. Campbell BK, Stark MJ. Psychopathology and personality characteristics in different forms of substance abuse. Int J Addict 1994; **25(12)**: 1467-74.
9. Fellows KW, Giannini AJ. Cinnamedryl: potential for abuse. J Toxicol: Clin Toxicol 1983; **20**: 93-97.
10. Dackis CA, Gold MS. Addictiveness of central stimulants. Adv Alcohol Subst Abuse 1990; **9(1-2)**: 9-26.
11. Hinsvark ON, Truant AP, Jenden BJ. Oral bioavailability and pharmokinetics of oral and resin bound forms of amphetamine and phentermine in man. J Pharmacolkinet Biopharm 1973; **1**: 319-339.
12. Catlin DH, Hatton CK. Use and abuse of anabolic and other drugs for athletic enhancement. Adv Intern Med 1991; **36**: 399-424.

CHAPTER 4

ANTICHOLINERGICS

The anticholinergics constitute a diverse group of compounds which share antagonism of muscarinic and atropinic cholinergic receptors as their unifying property. Anticholinergic compounds are usually obtained from botanicals, though discrete populations utilize over-the-counter prescription medications having anticholinergics properties. As diverse as the anticholinergics are in origin and type, they are equally diverse in effect. They can produce hallucinations, stimulation, increased sexual drive and feelings of euphoria. This class constitutes the most dangerous of the drugs of abuse since relatively small amounts can be fatal. Failure to recognize an acute anticholinergic toxicity may result in the death of the patient. Chronic to low to moderate level of anticholinergic abuse can produce serious but reversible changes.

LABORATORY TESTING

The anticholinergics include a diverse group of legal and illicit pharmaceutical products, industrial compounds and botanicals. The physician should contact the reference laboratory for specific diagnostic protocols and procedures in each case.

HISTORY

The anticholinergics have a long history in Western Civilization. In pharaonic Egypt, deadly nightshade, *Atropa belladonna*, was used as an eye drop preparation to induce mydriasis in women. This produced the "black eyes" which were then considered a sign of beauty. This fashion was continued throughout the Roman Empire, Middle Ages and Renaissance. It was during the Middle Ages that belladonna received it name. It comes from the Italian words meaning "beautiful woman."

There is evidence that during these historical periods, overdoses of belladonna were also used as a poison. Dio Cassius records gossip that Livia, the wife of Caesar Augustus, and Agrippina, the mother of Nero, utilized this anticholinergic compound to dispose of rival claimants for their sons' hold on the Roman Imperial throne. During the Renaissance, it was common but probably false knowledge that Lucrezia Borgia wore a ring which carried belladonna to poison the enemies of her brother, Cesare, and their father, Pope Alexander.[1]

Another popular Renaissance atropinic poison was aconite, a plant related to the buttercup. It was this poison which killed Romeo in William Shakespeare's *Romeo and Juliet*, and was mentioned in the troubadour poetry of Bertran de Born.[2]

The European mandrake (*mandragora*) is an anticholinergic plant with a history as equally colorful as that of belladonna. It was used as a poison, love potion, medium of wizardry, somnolent, facilitator of pregnancy and a panacea. In the Medieval European era, mandrake was in short supply because of overutilization due to its supposed connection to the spirits of the dark. According to learned customs, it could be safely harvested only by prescribed ritual. In this ritual, prayers were said over the plant under the light of a full moon. It was then uprooted by a black dog attached to the plant by a red or black cord. The human harvesters filled their ears with wax because it was believed that when the mandrake was pulled from the ground, it uttered a shriek which inflicted insanity to those unfortunate enough to hear it. In the Renaissance, it was documented erroneously that mandrake grew prolifically on the ground below the gallows. Leonardo da Vinci, in an attempt to utilize the scientific method, hypothesized that mandrake grew from the semen of the condemned men as it spurted forth during their death throes.[3]

Henbane and wolfsbane, both members of the *Hyoscyamus* family, were associated with satanic powers. Henbane was utilized in satanic rites and secular orgies from the Medieval era to modern times. During the Medieval era, it was mixed with semen, urine, menstrual blood, turnip and occasionally feces, and ground to a paste. It was then baked in the form of a satanic eucharistic host.[4] Henbane was another favorite poison of Shakespeare's, and it was the poison used to kill Hamlet's father.

At ultra low doses, wolfsbane can give increased energy and demonic savagery to troops. It was probably used by the armies of Walachian princeling Vlad Tepas (Vlad the Impalir).[5] Because of the bat which figured on his coat of arms ("drakul" in medieval Romanian), legends of nearby Transylvania, and the fertile imagination of the Irish novelist Bram Stoker, wolfsbane is now forever associated with the legend of the vampire, Count Dracula and Nosferatu as well as of the Wolfman.[5]

Datura and asthmador are two New World botanicals with atropinic properties. Asthmador (genus *Lobelia*) was adopted by American pioneers who observed Native Americans drying and smoking this plant. As a result, it was named "Indian tobacco." Currently, this bush-like plant is used as a border in home gardens and is readily available throughout the United States. It is used as a natural tea in health food stores and as a substitute for tobacco in "natural cigarettes." Previously it was used in Nicoban® and other tobacco substitutes to help people stop smoking. It is currently available as a home remedy in Western Pennsylvania, Eastern Ohio and the Appalachian regions. As a home remedy, it can be used an emetic, carminative, abortifacient, appetite stimulant and "digestive."[6]

The *Datura* genus includes the jimson weed and the thorn apple. The former plant, also known as "loco weed," was used by the Yaqui and other Mexican Native American tribes for ritualistic purposes. It was used on cattle drives by the cowboys and wranglers of the Old West to reduce boredom and enhance endurance. It is thought that some of the more bizarre outlaws of that time such as Johnny Ringo were chronic abusers of the jimson weed.[7]

In the latter half of the twentieth century, commercial sources of over-the-counter drugs containing diphenhydramine, meclizine, scopolamine, hyoscyamine and atropine are sources for anticholinergic activity. In addition to its direct effects, an anticholinergic/antihistaminic synergizes the euphoriant effects of opiates. It is therefore often used by addicts as a "booster" when heroin and morphine are in short supply.

POPULATION AT RISK

The populations abusing anticholinergics vary according to the effect which is sought. Low doses may be used as a euphoriant by one group while a second group uses higher doses to obtain hallucinogenic effects.

The most popular of the large number of anticholinergics available is trihexyphenidyl. This drugs accounts for approximately 75 percent of all anticholinergic drug abuse. It is a much sought-after drug in the jails and prisons of the United States, Canada and Great Britain. Outside prisons, it can also be used as an adulterant for LSD.[8]

Asthmador is generally used in Appalachia as a home remedy and its use is generally limited to those in isolated rural or mountainous communities. Approximately 10 percent of the population of upper Appalachia has used asthmador at least once. Asthmador has also experienced a recent resurgence as a "natural" and legal euphoriant and hallucinogen. This renaissance of asthmador seems to be limited to individuals between the ages of twenty and fifty.[9]

Wolfsbane, henbane and the related fleabane are still used in satanic rituals in the United States. The demographic profile of these users tends to be literate high-school graduates of both sexes, although the males predominate. Generally these patrons are from small towns or isolated subpockets in large urban communities. Their religious training tends to be Protestant in background, and the racial composition is overwhelmingly caucasian.[8]

Schizophrenic patients are a major source of abusers since they are often prescribed such anticholinergic agents as Cogentin®, Akineton® and Benadryl®. Generally they utilize these drugs to overcome the negative symptoms of their illness. It has been noted in the literature that when schizophrenics discontinue their neuroleptic medication, they tend to continue taking their anticholinergics in amounts in excess of those prescribed. The advent of newer neuroleptics that act at alpha-dopaminergic and serotonergic receptors (such as amprozide, clozapine, risperidone and seroquel) will probably end the rationale for prescribing anticholinergics to schizophrenics. These newer neuroleptic medications have few extrapyramidal side effects and, unlike the traditional neuroleptics, they act to ameliorate the negative symptoms of schizophrenia.[10]

PHYSIOLOGY AND BIOCHEMISTRY

Anticholinergic drugs act by antagonizing muscarinic and nicotinic cholinergic receptors. Muscarinic receptors are found centrally in the reticular activating system, the basal ganglia, and the limbic system. They are also found in the projection of the nucleus basalis of Meynert, to the basal and horizontal layers of the cortex. Peripherally, they are found at the postganglionic receptors of the parasympathetic nervous system.

There are two kinds of muscarinic receptors. The presynaptic M2 autoreceptors are associated with increased activity of the potassium channels. The postsynaptic M1 receptors are associated with decreased potassium activity. The nicotinic receptors are centrally distributed in the spinal cord, cerebral cortex, and some subcortical areas. Peripherally, they are found at the preganglionic neurosynapses and the skeletal motor endplate.

Botanicals contain one or more of three major types of anticholinergic compounds: lobeline, atropine (hyoscyamine), and scopolamine. Lobeline is a substitute piperidine compound which is water soluble. It acts on both muscarinic and nicotinic receptors. Centrally and peripherally it can agonize sympathetic receptors or antagonize parasympathetic receptors on the respective ganglia. It stimulates cholinergic activity in small doses but depresses it in larger doses. In addition to activity at cholinergic sites, it also has dopaminergic agonist activity, although the specific dopaminergic subsites have not yet been determined.[11]

Atropine is also called hyoscyamine. It is the organic ester formed by the combination of tropic acid and tropine. Atropine produces multiple effects at many organ systems. Centrally, it inhibits cholinergic receptors in the reticular activating substance, producing excitation. Cholinergic inhibition in the medulla oblongata produces decreased respiration leading to respiratory arrest at higher doses. In the peripheral nervous system, it can produce tremors which are a function of myoneural pathology. It acts upon the iris to dilate the pupil (mydriasis) and the ciliary muscle to inhibit accommodation (cycloplegia) producing photosensitivity and presbyopia.

In the cardiovascular system, most effects are produced by competitive inhibition of the vagus. Atropine blocks regulation by the sino-atrial node. As a result, there is tachycardia which leads progressively to atrial arrhythmia, widening of the QRS complex and A-V dissociation. While atropine produces minimal effects on blood pressure, the mechanism causing the characteristic flushed skin is unknown. In the respiratory system, there is decreased bronchial dilation due to inhibition of bronchial and bronchiolar smooth muscle tone.[12]

The only consistent endocrine effect of atropine is increased release of antidiuretic hormones. In the genitourinary tract, there is possible diminished ovulation. Increased tubular reabsorption is probably a function of atropinic-mediated effects on ADH secretion. The effects upon smooth muscle tissue produces dilation of the bladder, urethra and renal calyces.

In the digestive tract, atropine decreases gastric secretion. There is diminished release of amylase and partial inhibition of histamine-dependent hydrochloric acid release. Peristalsis is diminished in the small and large intestines which, in the large intestine, can progress to complete paralysis. While there is consistent antiperistalsis in the gallbladder, the choledochal sphincter can be constricted or relaxed by atropine.[13]

Scopolamine acts in a generally similar fashion as atropine but there are distinctive differences. Scopolamine is an organic ester formed by the combination of tropic acid and scopine. Its effects on the central nervous system are the mirror image of atropine. At low doses, it produces a characteristic twilight sleep with an amnestic period. In moderate doses, there is drowsiness or dreamless sleep associated with reduced REM phase. Higher doses produce excitation or irritability. Scopolamine's effects upon the eye are similar to that of atropine but much more intense. In addition, scopolamine acts on the macula of the utricle and saccule of the labyrinthine vestibules. In this manner, it decreases sensitivity to most forms of repetitive motion including pitch yaws, sway and tumble.

Scopolamine's effects on the cardiovascular system, gastrointestinal system and respiratory tract are less intense and of shorter duration than those of atropine. Otherwise they are similar.

All of the anticholinergic compounds are readily absorbed through the gastrointestinal tract and mucosa. There is also a very limited absorption through the eye and the skin. Gastrointestinal absorption occurs at the rate of 25 percent, with rapid distribution throughout the body. Effects are experienced within one hour. Metabolism is hepatic with sulfonation and hydrogenation being the most common pathways. Approximately 50 percent of atropine, 75 percent of lobeline and 90 percent of scopolamine are metabolized. All three cross the placental barrier but do not affect respiration of the fetus at term. Neither of these drugs interfere with uterine contractions during birth (see Table 4-1).

MEDICAL COMPLICATIONS

In anticholinergic intoxication, several potential complications exist, all of which are potentially lethal. Competitive inhibition at the motor end-plate produces relative paralysis of smooth muscle. Competitive inhibition also releases control of the sinoatrial node, producing tachycardia which can lead to atrial arrhythmias, widening of the QRS, atrioventricular dissociation and eventually asystole.

Drying of the mucus membranes can produce xerostomia. Photosensitivity produced by mydriasis can secondarily enhance the restlessness, irritability and disorientation of the intoxicated anticholinergic patient.

Table 4-1: Commonly Available Anticholinergic Sources in the U.S.

Type	Agent	
Antidepressants	Amitriptyline	Imipramine
	Amoxapine	Maprotiline
	Desipramine	Nortriptyline
	Doxepin	Trimipramine
Antihistamines	Antozoline	Diphenhydramine
	Benzotropine	Hydroxyzine
	Biperidin	Ketamedrin
	Bonine	Meclizine
	Barbinoxamine	Procyclidine
	Cyclizine	Tripelennamine
	Cyproheptadine	Trihexyphenidyl
Antimuscarinics	Adiphenine	Oxyphencyclimine
	Anisotropine	Mepenzolate
	Glycopyrrolate	Triphenamil
	Hexocyclium	Tropicamide
Antispasmodics	Atropine sulfate	Lobeline
	Hyoscyamine	Scopolamine
Botanicals	Angel's trumpet	Fleabane
	Asthmador	Fly agaric
	Balladonna	Henbane
	Choke cherry	Jimson weed
	Deadly nightshade	Kinnikinnick
	Datura	Luco weed
	Dogbane	Nutmeg
	European mandrake	Thorn apple
	Wolfbane	
Ganglionic Blocking Agents	Hexamethonium	Pentolinium
	Mecamylamine	Trimethaphen
Illicit Sources	Phencyclidine	
Phenothizines	Chlorpromazine	Promethizine
	Mesoridazine	Thioridazine

In more than a few cases, naive patients have utilized jimson weed, deadly nightshade and thorn apple without pharmaceutical intent. Nightshade has a bitter taste which makes it a pungent addition to salad. Jimson weed tastes somewhat bitter and is aromatic and not altogether unpleasant. Medical complications do not tend to occur in anticholinergic withdrawal.

DIAGNOSIS

The classic presentation of the anticholinergic abuser was provided nearly a century ago by Sir William Osler. These patients present "mad as a hatter, red as a beet, and dry as a bone." This aphorism distinctly and colorfully describes the dry flushed skin and the disorientation of the intoxicated patient.

There generally tend to be complaints of an inability to urinate or of burning in the urethra. There is dysphagia, constipation and hoarseness. Patients note photosensitivity, diplopia, visual hallucinations and body-image distortions. Upon examination, these patients tend to be easily distractible and garrulous. Blood pressure may be normal or decreased in the presence of tachycardia. Scopolamine intoxication differs from atropinic and lobelinic toxicity by the presence of somnolence, possible bradycardia, bilateral Babinski sign, and minimal flushing of the skin.[14-17]

TREATMENT

The most serious problems are the central effects, ileus and atonic bladder. Methacholine, pilocarpine and physostigmine salicylate all reverse peripheral symptomatology. Physostigmine has the additional benefit in that it crosses the blood brain barrier, reversing both central and peripheral effects. Physostigmine inhibits the cholinesterase-induced breakdown of acetylcholine. Some authors recommend against the use of physostigmine since it is associated with increased bronchial secretions and, rarely, asystole. However, careful familiarization with this antidote can make it a valuable product.[18]

Generally, physostigmine is given in dosages of 1 mg. to 2 mg., intramuscularly or intravenously. It is usually employed to reverse the effects of ileus, atonic bladder and cardiac arrhythmias. Because of the anticholinergic effects on the heart, continuous EKG monitoring should be instituted. If the widening of the QRS increases beyond 10 mm, or AV dissociation appears, or there is evidence of arrhythmias, physostigmine should be given every 20 minutes until the irregularity disappears. In maintaining the patient with physostigmine, it should be noted that physostigmine is completely metabolized within 90 to 120 minutes. At that time, an additional 0.5 mg. to 2 mg. should be administered.

Because of the depression of the medulla oblongata, the treatment area should have the capability to maintain artificial respiration. Delirium and disorientation also respond to physostigmine.

Because of dryness of the corneal surface, the patient should be checked for contact lenses and these should be removed if present. The surface of the cornea can be moistened with methylcellulose solutions and the mucous membranes with saline.

Anhydrosis is generally treated with 0.6 N saline solution intravenously at a rate of 100 cc to 120 cc per hour. Because of mydriasis, these particular procedures should be performed in a darkened room.

If ingestion is within two hours of treatment initiation, emesis can be induced with syrup of Ipecac. The patient should be intubated if he or she is convulsing. Gastric lavage can be performed with 60 mg. to 100 mg. of activated charcoal. Agitation generally responds to physostigmine salicylate. If there is no response, patients can be given lorazepam in 1 mg. to 2 mg. doses intramuscularly every hour in the absence of underlying pulmonary disease. If there is no response to lorazepam, then consider pentobarbital 100 mg. to 200 mg. intramuscularly or intravenously for an adult, or 25 mg. to 75 mg. for a child.

TYPICAL CASE PRESENTATION

The patient was a 37-year-old white male who presented to a community mental health center for evaluation. At that time, he was evaluated by the intake person and was observed to be "very agitated with pressured speech. He was very threatening." As a result, a psychiatrist was brought in on the case.

A mental status examination revealed pressured speech, labile affect and hyperkinetic behavior. He was disoriented to time only. Content was delusional with satanic references. Associations were loose. He could not or would not respond to tests of cognition. He admitted to visual hallucination of Lilliputian type as well as of "moving shadows." He told the examining psychiatrist, "I'm a schizophrenic, Dr. S- gives me pills but they're not working any more." A call was then placed to his treating psychiatrist.

While waiting for the return call a physical examination was conducted. His skin was found to be hot, dry and flushed. His pupils were dilated, conjunctivitis was present, fundi were within normal limits and there was sluggish response to accommodation. While examining the eyes, the patient described diplopia and photosensitivity. Pulse was rapid and weak. Bowel sounds were diminished and bladder was distended.

At this point, the diagnosis of anticholinergic intoxication was made. The patient, however, resisted therapy. He was restrained and treated with haloperidol 5 mg. intramuscularly. This was followed by physostigmine salicylate 2 mg. intramuscularly. The patient became less combative and a Foley catheter was introduced. A flat plate of the abdomen revealed ileus. A portable heart monitor revealed nonspecific arrhythmias and widening of the QRS interval. To relieve anhidrosis an IV line of 0.9 saline was run at 160 cc per hour. After a 20 minute interval, the physostigmine dosage was repeated.

Shortly thereafter, the patient was transferred by ambulance and under monitor to the nearest general hospital. There the dosage of physostigmine was repeated until the ileus and cardiac changes had been alleviated.

The treating psychiatrist called back and revealed that patient was a paranoid schizophrenic whom he treated with thiothixene 10 mg. four times a day, benztropine 1 mg. four times a day and diphenhydramine 50 mg. to 100 mg. at bedtime as needed. He denied knowledge of a previous history of anticholinergic psychosis. A follow-up examination of the patient revealed purchases of large amounts of diphenhydramine. In addition, the patient had received additional unauthorized refills of benztropine from a naive pharmacist to replace "lost medication."

An inpatient transfer to the hospital drug-rehabilitation unit was refused by the patient and his wife. Both, however, accepted the need for outpatient referral. He was referred for outpatient therapy to a psychiatrist familiar with dual diagnosis patients. To avoid his need for anticholinergics, risperidone was prescribed as his neuroleptic. He was also referred to an outpatient drug rehabilitation program.

NOTES

1.   Burchard J. Diarum 1483-1506. Paris: L. Thuane, 1883.
2.   Bonner W. Songs of the Troubadours. New York: St. Martin's Press, 1972.
3.   Taylor R. Leonardo of Florence. New York: MacMillan, 1927.
4.   Crump CG, Jacob EF. The Legacy of the Middle Ages. Oxford: Oxford University Press, 1926.

5. Purphilet J. Jeux et Sapience du Moyen Age. Paris: Thuane, 1940.

6. Cave K (ed.). The Diaries of Joseph Farrington. New Haven: Yale University Press, 1984.

7. Earp W. My Friend, Doc Holliday. New York: Nickleby, 1898.

8. Giannini AJ, Loiselle RH. Patterns of atropinic and anticholinergic drug abuse. (Research in progress.)

9. Goggin DA, Solomon GF. Trihexyphenidyl abuse for euphorigenic effect. Am J Psychiatry 1979; **136**:459-460.

10. Schifano F, di Costanzo E. Excessive use of anticholinergic drugs in a sub-sample of Italian schizophrenics. Int J Clin Pharmacol Ther Toxicol 1991; **29(5)**:184-6.

11. Goldstein JM. Seroquel: A potative atypical antipsychotic drug. J Clin Psychiatry 1995; **56(9)**:438-445.

12. Land W, Pinsky D, Salzman C. Abuse and misuse of anticholinergic medications. Hosp Community Psychiatry 1991; **42(6)**:580-1.

13. Castiglione F, Daniele B, Massacca G. Therapeutic strategy for the irritable bowel syndrome. Ital J Gastroenterol 1991; **23(8 Suppl 1)**:53-5.

14. Larson EW, Pfenning MA, Richelson E. Selectivity of antimuscarinic compounds for muscarinic receptors of human brain and heart. Psychopharmacology 1991; **103(2)**:162-5.

15. Hidalgo HA, Mowers RM. Anticholinergic drug abuse. DICP 1990; **24(1)**:40-1.

16. Warrens AN, Ron MA, Dawling S. Positive diagnosis of self-medication with homatropine eye drops. Br J Psychiatry 1990; **156**:124-5.

17. Flicker C, Serby M, Ferris SH. Scopolamine effects on memory, language, visuospatial praxis and psychomotor speed. Psychopharmacology 1990; **100(2)**:243-50.

18. Smilkstein MJ. As the pendulum swings: the saga of physostigmine. J Emer Med 1991; **9(4)**:275-7.

CHAPTER 5

BENZODIAZEPINES

Commonly called tranquilizers, the benzodiazepines are the most popularly prescribed psychotropic medication in the world. Since their introduction in 1960, they have consistently ranked in the top five of the most prescribed medications. They are generally prescribed as anxiolytics, soporifics and anticonvulsants.[1,2] In addition, they are inappropriately prescribed for the treatment of depression and for chemical restraint.[3,4] Benzodiazepines also have value on the street where they are used as recreational drugs. In the United States, they are sometimes used in combination with other drugs, although in Europe, they enjoy solo status.[5]

The benzodiazepines are totally synthetic compounds with no known analogues in nature. Generally they are manufactured throughout the world. In the United States the easy availability of benzodiazepines has precluded the establishment of illegal laboratories.

All benzodiazepines are usually obtained by prescription, legitimate or forged. They are easily available for potentially recreational use in sample form. It is estimated that nearly half of all street benzodiazepines come from physician samples.[6] Again because of easy availability, benzodiazepines are not "cut" or diluted. Tablets and capsules are the predominant form. Parenteral preparations are unusual[7,8,9] (see Table 5-1).

LABORATORY TESTING

Benzodiazepine levels can be obtained from either serum or urine samples. Nearly any of the available tests can be utilized. Thin layer chromatography has a role for qualitative analysis. For legal purposes, benzodiazepines should be tested by enzyme immunoassay (EIA) or gas chromatography/mass spectrometry (GC/MS). The former tests can be sensitive to 300 ng. per ml. and the latter to 100 ng. per ml. for either serum or urine samples. The benzodiazepines were generally longed-lived and they or their metabolites may be tested for 14 days. Each benzodiazepine usually has multiple active and inactive metabolites. In

Table 5-1: The Proprietary Benzodiazepines Available in the United States

Brand Name	Generic Name	Recommended Route of Administration
Ambien*	Zolpidem	p.o.
Ativan	Lorazepam	p.o., IV, IM
Dalmane	Flurazepam	p.o.
Halcion	Triazolam	p.o.
Klonopin	Clonazepam	p.o.
Libritab	Chlordiazepoxide	p.o.
Librium	Chlordiazepoxide	p.o., IV, IM
Librax	Chlordiazepoxide	p.o.
Restoril	Temazepam	p.o.
Serax	Oxazepam	p.o.
Tranxene	Chlorazepate	p.o.
Valium	Diazepam	p.o., IV
Xanax	Alprazolam	p.o.

*Non-benzodiazepine soporific with activity at B-Z receptors

testing for legal purposes or for "drug checks," the longest lived metabolite, active or inactive, as well as the parent compound, should be ordered for testing.[10-14]

HISTORY

The benzodiazepines were first synthesized in Switzerland in 1933, at Hoffmann-LaRoche laboratories. In the 1950's, they were compared to meperidine and found to have superior sedative properties.

In 1955, Earl Reader and Lee Sternback at Hoffman-LaRoche Laboratories in Switzerland synthesized chlordiazepoxide. Two years later, a series of experiments with a number of animal species under the direction of Lowell Randall and Wilhelm Schallek first noted the "taming" effects of chlordiazepoxide. Within three years, chlordiazepoxide, the prototypical benzodiazepine, was introduced for sale as Librium®. Within two years, diazepam (Valium®) was also sold by the same laboratory.

Benzodiazepines began replacing barbiturates, methaqualone and the other sedative-hypnotics as tranquilizers. It was soon discovered that halogenation of benzodiazepines increased soporific effects. Soon flurazepam, a fluorinated version of diazepam, was introduced as the first benzodiazepine "sleeping pill."

Valium® and Librium® are long-lived compounds with effects sometimes lasting several days. Over time, shorter acting benzodiazepines such as lorazepam and chlorazepate were introduced on the market. In the 1990's, the first ultra-short acting benzodiazepine, alprazolam (Xanax®), was introduced. It was soon followed by its halogenated soporific counterpart, triazolam (Halcion®).

In 1993, a novel tranquilizing compound was introduced. It was the sedating agent zolpidem (Ambien®). Although zolpidem does not structurally resemble benzodiazepines, it nevertheless has major activity at benzodiazepine receptors (B-Z receptors) and has similar clinical effects.

Benzodiazepines quickly became abused through misunderstanding and over-prescription by physicians as well as misuse by patients. There appeared in the 1960's a large subculture of frustrated housewives and over-stressed and over-extended career men and women totally dependent on tranquilizers. Their role in dealing with domestic angst was satirized in the Rolling Stones "Mother's Little Helper." Aldous Huxley who had described a compound "soma" with actions similar to benzodiazepines in his novel *Brave New World*, was alarmed at the latter compound's popularity. He then published *Brave New World Revisited* which advocated a rational use of tranquilizing and other psychoactive compounds. In the 1980's, Barbara Gordon published *I'm Dancing As Fast As I Can*. This autobiographical account chronicled the addiction and destruction of a highly creative personality.

Shortly thereafter, a spurious relationship between benzodiazepines and cancer was discovered. Although the association with cancer was never proven, fears about addiction, over-medication and lethality gradually developed.

POPULATIONS AT RISK

There are three high-risk populations for benzodiazepine addiction. These include those who receive over-prescribed amounts of benzodiazepines, those who abuse benzodiazepines as a sole drug, and those who abuse benzodiazepines in combination with other recreational drugs.

Those who receive over-prescribed benzodiazepines may obtain them from a single physician. More commonly, they obtain them from multiple physicians or from the supplies of other family members or friends. In this group, whites outnumber blacks and Asians, and females outnumber males, although exact reliable figures are not available.

It is worth noting that it is difficult in this group to actually assign the label of "addiction." Some authorities label as an addict any patient who utilizes benzodiazepines for four or more months. This ignores many clinical reasons for continuing benzodiazepines, such a petit mal epilepsy, panic disorder, generalized anxiety disorder and post traumatic stress disorder.

Benzodiazepines can also be bought on the street. This is generally an adolescent phenomenon. In this case, benzodiazepines may act as a gateway drug. The amount of solo abusers obtaining benzodiazepines through illicit sources comprise the smallest of the three groups.

Together, the people who use benzodiazepines as the sole or primary source of addiction constitute no more than 15 percent of all benzodiazepine abusers. The largest group of benzodiazepine addicts, 85 percent, use benzodiazepines in combination with other drugs. Nearly 20 to 40 percent of alcoholics and 25 to 50 percent of heroin and methadone addicts use benzodiazepines for the additive effect upon their primary drug of choice. Cocaine addicts, on the other hand, use benzodiazepines to come down more smoothly from a cocaine high. Approximately 10 to 25 percent of cocaine addicts use benzodiazepines for this purpose.

Although amphetamines have a similar effect to cocaine, most amphetamine addicts use benzodiazepines in a slightly different manner. They generally use amphetamine to "rev up" in the morning and benzodiazepines to "come down" in the evening. This combined use of uppers and downers comprises approximately 30 percent of all amphetamine addicts.[15] Benzodiazepines are generally not used in combination with marijuana, phencyclidine, psychedelics, steroids or volatiles.[16]

CHEMISTRY AND PHYSIOLOGY

Benzodiazepines act through gamma-aminobutyric acid (GABA receptors). GABA receptors are the most common of all inhibitory receptors. The GABA receptor is a large complex. It includes a GABA receptor site and "B-P" receptor site, which is acted upon by the sedative-hypnotics, and a "B-Z" receptor site, which is acted upon by the benzodiazepines. These separate receptor sites act to gate chloride channels. Although the benzodiazepines have a weak effect upon these channels, they have an additive effect on GABA to greatly increase the permeability of the chloride channels. The benzodiazepines do so by increasing the frequency of channel openings. The sedative-hypnotics in contradistinction act either independently or in accompaniment with GABA to increase the duration in which the chloride channels remain in a "open" state.

Because sedative-hypnotics have some independent action and they increase the duration of opening, they are referred to as "direct" receptors. Since the activity of benzodiazepines is dependent upon the presence of GABA, and since the action is dependent upon frequency rather than duration of openings, the B-Z receptors are referred to as "co-receptors."[17,18,19,20]

There are two types of B-Z receptors: the "B-Z 1" and the "B-Z 2." The benzodiazepines work upon both of these.[21] The benzodiazepines work at many sites in the brain, some of which have been hypothesized to produce a specific action. Activity in the medulla is thought to affect neuromuscular action, while activity of the cerebellum produces modulation of the same action and reduces intention tremors.

Anxiolytic effects are thought to be produced at the frontal cortex and hippocampus. Physiologic tremors are reduced by activity at the neuromuscular junction. GABA sites in the substantia nigra reduce resting tremors and modulate motor activity. Activity at the superior colliculi is associated with visual and sensory arousal. Activity in the zona reticulata antagonizes a general arousal state.[22]

In addition to the above specific effects, there are general actions of all benzodiazepines. These usually affect electroencephalograms by increasing fast beta activity, decreasing amplitude, and diminishing stage four sleep.[23-26]

Normal, uncomplicated addiction is associated with decreased respiratory rate and decreased blood pressure. There may be decreased left ventricular stroke work with resulting tachycardia and diminished cardiac output. These latter effects are minor. Although benzodiazepines have an indication for muscle relaxation, many researchers have questioned the existence of this particular action.

As a group, the absorption, half-life and duration of activity differs widely (see Table 5-2). The individual drugs vary from very short-lived, such as alprazolam with a half-life of 11 hours, to chlordiazepoxide with a half-life of 2 days. The variable half-life is useful clinically as a criterion for different clinical applications. The drug elimination times are

Table 5-2: Pharmacological Data, Benzodiazepine (Oral Forms Only)

Benzodiazepine	Half-Life	Peak Serum Levels
Alprazolam	11 hrs.	1-2 hrs.
Chlordiazepoxide	24-48 hrs.	2-3 hrs.
Clonazepam	18-48 hrs.	2 hrs.
Diazepam	72 hrs.	1 hr.
Flurazepam	2 hrs.	5-1 hr.
Lorazepam	12 hrs.	2 hrs.
Oxazepam	8 hrs.	3 hrs.
Temazepam	9 hrs.	1.5 hrs.
Triazolam	3.5 hrs.	2 hrs.

also different. The pattern is biphasic for all members of this group. There is an initial fast phase measured in hours, followed by a slow elimination phase usually measured in days. Most benzodiazepines have active metabolites. Metabolites are usually dimethylated or glucuronide forms, although some such as chlordiazepoxide have lactim metabolites.[27,28,29]

MEDICAL COMPLICATIONS

The benzodiazepines are among the safest of all recreational drugs as well as all prescribed drugs. Death usually occurs only in combination, although a report 20 years ago measured the lethality of a single dosage in excess of 700 mg.[30] A Canadian study of benzodiazepine deaths found that they occurred predominantly in combination with alcohol or propoxyphene. Various American studies identified mortality only in combination with alcohol, opiates or sedative-hypnotics.[31-33]

Long-term addiction may be associated with paradoxical anxiety or agitation. There are also frequent reports of ataxia, headaches, constipation, diplopia and insomnia. Many patients, especially in summer months, report photosensitivity associated with a rash. This rash may occur only in areas of high contact such as underneath the bra, brief or panty elastic bands. Incontinence and disruption of the ovulatory cycle occur in a few patients. Agranulocytosis is rare but is a potentially fatal side effect. Although hiccoughs are a rare and non-dangerous side effect, their cause should be recognized in long-term benzodiazepine use.[34,35]

Table 5-3: Dosage Conversion Table for Benzodiazepines

Alprazolam	1 mg.
Chlordiazepoxide	25 mg.
Clonazepam	4 mg.
Clorazepate	15 mg.
Diazepam	10 mg.
Flurazepam	15 mg.
Holazepam	40 mg.
Lorazepam	2 mg.
Oxazepam	10 mg.
Temazepam	15 mg.
Triazolam	1 mg.
Zolpidem*	20 mg.

*Non-benzodiazepine soporific with activity at B-Z receptors.

TREATMENT

In cases of benzodiazepine overdose, direct intervention is seldom necessary. It is important, however, to support respiration and blood pressure. If respiration falters, it can be initially treated with administration of pure oxygen. If this is ineffective, respiration must be supported.

Hypotension can be treated with 0.9 N saline intravenously at a rate of 80-120 cc per hour. If necessary, norepinephrine can be added to the IV bottle at a concentration of 4 ampuls per 250 cc saline solution. Norepinephrine should be titrated against blood pressure.

Benzodiazepine addiction can be treated on an inpatient or on an outpatient basis. Inpatient treatment is usually necessary only in cases of extremely high dosages, impaired physical status, or polydrug abuse. Because of some risk of seizure, the patient should be placed on seizure precautions.[36] After the first 12 to 24 hours, propranolol is administered at a rate of 20 mg. to 40 mg. every 6 to 8 hours and is gradually decreased over a 3 to 6 day period.[37] In cases of co-existing diabetes mellitus, idiopathic bradycardia, or idiopathic hypertension, propranolol is contraindicated. As an alternative, lorazepam can be utilized as a withdrawal agent. The total daily dosage is based upon equivalence with the particular benzodiazepine abused (see Table 5-3). The daily dosage of lorazepam should be divided into every 8 hours to every 6 hours. In the case of propranolol, detoxification can be completed within 4 to 6 days; with lorazepam, 3 to 5 days.[38,39]

If detoxification is attempted on an outpatient basis, the daily dosage of the particular abused benzodiazepine should be reduced by 10 percent per day each week. The patient should be seen on a twice-weekly basis and his or her condition monitored. If symptoms of anxiety appear as a result of the withdrawal state, hydroxyzine or propranolol can be used to ameliorate the anxiety as well as other physical symptoms.

TYPICAL CASE PRESENTATION

The patient was a 49-year-old Asian male who presented to the emergency room at 2:30 a.m. because he said he lost his prescription. He claimed to be receiving Valiums for "a nervous condition." A telephone call was placed by the triage nurse to his physician. A return call was made by the family practitioner who was providing coverage for the patient's doctor who had been on vacation for four days and was not expected to return for six days. The doctor did not know the patient and could not provide a further history. The triage nurse then referred the case to the psychiatric resident.

The resident examined the patient, who told her he had been receiving Valium for three years at the current dosage and for four previous years at a lower dosage. He said "I have nerves, I can't work without the Valium." He was a draftsman for a local architectural firm and had no work-related problems. He denied abuse of Valium, alcohol or other drugs.

Examination, however, revealed an elevated temperature of 99.6°F and a pulse of 90 beats/min. His speech was pressured, his behavior hyperkinetic and his demeanor hyperirritable. There was a moderate resting tremor. Nystagmus was present in the horizontal plane. Romberg's sign was present.

During the examination, the patient said "I'm desperate. I take about twelve Valium a day." He then admitted to "doctor shopping" to maintain his benzodiazepine addiction. He agreed to be admitted for detoxification. A GC/MS confirmed his dosage history.

After admission to the detoxification unit, he was placed on "bed rest and bathroom privileges with assistance only." Seizure precautions were instituted. Blood pressure was stable at 125/90 mm Hg. Detoxification was initiated with lorazepam 4 mg. every 6 hours by mouth. The patient was mildly uncomfortable but vital signs were stable and tremors did not increase in intensity. It was therefore decided not to add propranolol.

Dosage of lorazepam was decreased by 1 mg. every other day. On the tenth day of withdrawal, the patient became extremely uncomfortable, coarse tremors were visible and pulse rate increased to 94 beats per min. At this point, propranolol 40 mg. five times a day was prescribed to good effect. He was then detoxified without incident.

After detoxification, the patient was treated on an inpatient rehabilitation unit. Here his underlying generalized anxiety disorder as well as his addiction were addressed. After three weeks of inpatient therapy, he was referred to a psychiatrist familiar with dual diagnosis patients as well as a Narcotics Anonymous and a local panic/phobia/anxiety self-help group. His anxiety was treated with a serotonin reuptake inhibitor (SRI) rather than a benzodiazepine.

NOTES

1. Tsoi WV. Insomnia: drug treatment. Ann Acad Med Singapore 1991; **20(2)**:269-72.
2. Matuzas W, Jack E. The drug treatment of panic disorder. Psychiatr Med 1991; **9(2)**:215-43.
3. Doherty MH. Benzodiazepine sedation in critically ill patients. AACN Clin Issues Crit Care Nurs 1991; **32(4)**:748-63.
4. Billig N, Cohen-Mansfield J, Lipson S. Pharmacological treatment of agitation in a nursing home. J Am Geriatri Soc 1991; **39(10)**:1002.
5. Strang J, Griffiths P, Abbey J, Gossop M. Survey of use of injected benzodiazepine among drug users in Britain. BMJ 1994; **308(6936)**:1082.
6. Giannini AJ, Loiselle RM. Patterns of benzodiazepine use and abuse. (Not yet submitted.)
7. Rastergar DA. Drug dealers. Arch Fam Med 1995; **4(7)**:576.
8. Rosser WW. Anxiety of benzodiazepines. Can Fam Physician 1995; **41**:760, 763-5, 772-6.
9. WHO Expert Committee on drug dependence. World Health Organ Tech Rep Ser 1991; **808**:i-iv, 1-20.
10. Moore CM, Sato K, Satsumata Y. Rapid monitoring of benzodiazepines in clinical samples by using on-line column switching HPLC. Clin Chem 1991; **37(6)**:804-8.

11. Seno H, Suzuki O, Kumazawa T, Hattori H. Rapid isolation with Sep-Pak C18 cartridges and wide-bore capillary gas chromatography of benzophenones, the acid-hydrolysis products of benzodiazepines. J Anal Toxicol 1991; **15(1)**:21-4.

12. Needleman SB, Porvaznik M. Identification of parent benzodiazepines by gas chromatography/mass spectroscopy (GC/MS from urinary extracts treated with B-glucuronidase. Forensic Sci Int 1995; **73(1)**:49-60.

13. Meatherall R. Benzodiazepine screening using EMIT II and TDx: urine hydrolysis pretreatment required. J Anal Toxicol 1994; **18(7)**:385-90.

14. Ensing K, Bosman IJ, Ebgerts AC, Franke JP, de Zeeuw RA. Application of radioreceptor assays for systematic toxicological analysis—1. Procedures for radioreceptor assays for antihistaminics, anticholinergics and benzodiazepines. J Pharm Biomed Anal 1994; **12(1)**:53-8.

15. Food and Drug Administration. Benzodiazepines: Extent of Use, Abuse and Misuse. Washington, D.C.: U.S. Government Printing Office, 1981.

16. Hawley CJ, Tattersall M, Dellaportas C, Hallstrom C. Comparison of long-term benzodiazepines users in three settings. Br J Psychiatry 1994; **165(6)**:792-6.

17. Ku TW, Miller WH, Bondinell WE, Erhard KF, Keenan RM, Nichols AJ, Peishoff CE, Samanen JM, Wong AS, Huffman WF. Potent non-peptide fibrinogen receptor antagonists which present an alternative pharmacophore. J Med Chem 1995; **38(1)**:9-12.

18. Mihic SJ, Whiting PJ, Klein RL, Wafford KA, Harris RA. A single amino acid of the human gamma-aminobutyric acid type A receptor gamma 2 subunit determines benzodiazepine efficacy. J Biol Chem 1994; **269(52)**:468-773.

19. Maggio R, Barbier P, Bolognesi ML, Minarini A, Tedeschi D, Melchiorre C. Binding profile of the selective muscarinic receptor antagonist tripitramine. Eur J Pharmacol 1994; **268(3)**:459-62.

20. Sanger DJ, Benavides J, Perrault G, Morel E, Cohen C, Joly D. Zivkovic B. Recent developments in the behavioral pharmacology of benzodiazepine (omega) receptors: evidence for the functional significance of receptor subtypes. Science 1974; **145**:534-535.

21. Wieland HA, Luddens H. Four amino acid exchanges convert a diazepam-insensitive, inverse agonist-preferring GABAA receptor into a diazepam-preferring GABAA receptor. J Med Chem 1994; **37(260)**:4576-80.

22. Izquierdo I, Medine JH. GABAA receptor modulation of memory: the role of endogenous benzodiazepines. Trends Pharmacol Sci 1991; **12(7)**:260-5.

23. Fraser DD, Mudrick-Donnon La, MacVicar BA. Astrocytic GABA receptors. Glia 1994; **11(2)**:83-93.

24. Durbin CG Jr. Sedation in the critically ill patient. New Horiz 1994; **2(1)**:640-674.

25. Medina JH, Paladini AC, Izquierdo I. Naturally occurring benzodiazepines and benzodiazepine-like molecules in brain. Behav Brain Res 1993; **58(1-2)**:1-8.

26. Medine JH, Peña C, Piva M, Wolfman C, De Stein ML, Wasowski C, Da Cunha C, Izquierdo I, Paladina AC. Benzodiazepines in the brain. Their origin and possible biological roles. Mol Neurobiol 1992; **6(4)**:377-8.

27. Eadie MJ. Formation of active metabolites of anticonvulsant drugs. A review of their pharmacokinetic and therapeutic significance. Clin Pharmacokinet 1991; **21(1)**:27-41.

28. Bailey L, Ward M, Musa MN. Clinical pharmacokinetics of benzodiazepines. J Clin Pharmacol 1994; **34(8)**:804-11.

29. Longmire AW, Seger DL. Topics in clinical pharmacology; flumazenil, a benzodiazepine antagonists. Am J Med Sci 1993; **306(1)**:49-52.

30. Detre TP, Jarecki HG. Modern Psychiatric Treatment. Philadelphia: J.B. Lippincott and Co., 1971; 183-184.

31. Sellers EM, Ciraulo DA, DuPont RL, Griffiths RR, Kosten TR, Romach MK, Woody GE. Alprazolam and benzodiazepine dependence. J Clin Psychiatry 1993; **54(Supple)**:64-75.

32. Spivey WH, Roberts Jr, Derlet RW. A clinical trial of escalating doses of flumazenil for reversal of suspected benzodiazepines overdose in the emergency department. Ann Emerg Med 1993; **22(12)**:1813-21.

33. Salzman C. Issues and controversies regarding benzodiazepine use. NIDA Res Monogr 1993; **131**:68-88.

34. Gudex C. Adverse effects of benzodiazepines. Soc Sci Med 1991; **33(5)**:587-96.

35. The Use of Benzodiazepine Hypnotics: A Scientific Examination of a Clinical Controversy. Proceeding of a roundtable symposium. Phoenix, Arizona, April 10, 1992.

36. Watson C. Status epilepticus. Clinical features, pathophysiology and treatment. West J Med 1991; **155(6)**:626-31.

37. Neff DA, McQueen KD. Beta-blockers in alcohol withdrawal. DICP 1991; **25(1)**:31-2.

38. Morrison J. Withdrawal from tranquilizers. Practitioner 1991; **235(1506)**:684, 687-8.

39. Philip BK. Drug reversal: Benzodiazepine receptors and antagonists. J Clin Anesth 1993; 5(Suppl 1):46S-51S.

CHAPTER 6

COCAINE

Cocaine is one of the most popular drugs in America. It is predominantly used in four different forms. The least-used form, coca paste, is derived directly from the coca leaf and smoked.

Ether is used to process coca paste into cocaine hydrochloride, the "powder" form of cocaine. Powdered cocaine is generally snorted. It produces a fast "rush" but its popularity is limited by its high price. Cocaine hydrochloride is seen as an elite drug and it is not commonly used in middle and lower economic groups.

Derivatives of cocaine hydrochloride include "free base" and "crack." Both of these latter forms are an alkaline base. Freebase cocaine uses ether, where crack uses hydroxides or baking soda to accomplish this task. Base forms of cocaine are usually smoked alone or with heroin (boy-girl) or with phencyclidine (space-base).[1] They provide an immediate rush but are of shorter duration and action. The base forms of cocaine tend to be much more addicting than cocaine hydrochloride.[2,3]

LABORATORY TESTING

Cocaine or its metabolites may have their presence tested in either the serum or urine. Major inactive metabolites of cocaine are benzoylecgonine and ecgonine methyl ester. Norcocaine is an active metabolite.[4]

A urine sample obtained from a cocaine user breaks down to 30 to 40 percent benzoylecgonine, 25 to 50 percent ecgonine methyl ester and 10 percent unchanged cocaine. Since the ecgonine metabolites are formed by esterification, serum cholinesterase must be deactivated in the samples. This can be accomplished by use of physostigmine or a fluoride inhibitor. Generally, benzoylecgonine, the longest-lived metabolite with a half-life of approximately six hours, is usually assayed. Most commonly used techniques include thin-layer chromatography, radioimmunoassay, gas chromatography/mass spectrometry and high pressure liquid chromatography. Utilizing the latter three methods, benzoylecgonine can be detected in the urine up to six days after the last use of cocaine.[5-10]

HISTORY

Coca leaves were first used within the North Central areas of South America from 3 to 4 thousand years ago. Leaves were chewed by various pre-Columbian civilizations. Apparently some of these groups chewed the leaves with ashes, an early form of crack cocaine.

With the emergence of the Incan civilization, coca was utilized as a sacramental drug by the priest and warrior classes. In addition, the armies of the Inca chewed coca leaves to ward off hunger, thirst, fatigue and fear.

The Spanish conquistadors under Francisco Pizarro apparently discovered cocaine by experimenting with it on a sporadic basis. In the Napoleonic period, cocaine was adopted by the upper and middle classes in Europe as a recreational and medicinal compound. Medically, it was utilized as a local anesthetic, a use which still continues.

Throughout the nineteenth century, various tinctures of cocaine were sold as alcoholic beverages throughout Europe. The most popular of these was Vin Mariani in which cocaine powder was dissolved in Italian wine. It was well received throughout the world and carried endorsements by notable figures of the day including Pope Leo, the Prince of Wales and U.S. President William McKinley. An American version was a carbonated cocaine beverage, Coca-Cola®. These refreshments continued to be sold until the passage of the Harrison Narcotic Act in 1905. After declining use during the Prohibition Era, cocaine enjoyed a resurgence in the 1930's, occasioning Cole Porter to write "I get no kick from cocaine; mere alcohol doesn't thrill me at all, but I get a kick out of you."

Cocaine remained an elite drug due to its great expense. In the 1970's, however, a phenomenon occurred that would make cocaine a drug of the masses. At that time, Peruvian peasants began manufacturing a free-base form of coca paste with ether. This was the original "free-base," called that because the base cocaine was freed. Free-base appeared in California in about 1974. A large ritual developed around it because various chemicals, glass pipes and extraction kits were needed to use it. Cocaine was mixed with ether, heated with a pipe and the vapors inhaled.

Popular experimentation with free-base slowed when one set session literally exploded in the face of comedian, Richard Pryor. His resulting burn injuries and critical condition greatly reduced the popularity of this form of cocaine.

In the late 1970's and early 1980's, underground chemists in the Netherlands Antilles began modifying coca paste with baking soda and rum to form "base-rock" or "Roxanne," i.e., crack cocaine. By 1983, base rock was being shipped from the Southern Caribbean and Latin America through the Bahamas. Within a year, crack cocaine was introduced to the U.S.[11,12]

In the latter phase of the Reagan presidency, the White House Drug Policy Office under Dr. Carlton Turner devised the initial government response to the increased use and trafficking of cocaine by gangs. During the Bush presidency, this policy was further elaborated and the "zero tolerance approach" was adopted. In this program, even trace amounts of cocaine were not tolerated, and anyone found with small amounts of cocaine in his or her possession was immediately prosecuted. Money was given to South American countries to eradicate the coca bush and pay farmers to plant alternative crops. This effort, which was coordinated by the Drug Enforcement Administration, sought to stop cocaine at its source. Within the U.S., additional penalties were levied for the sale of cocaine in the schoolyard or to school children. Confiscatory legislation was passed that enabled DEA agents to seize the property of drug lords as well as street dealers. The U.S. Information Agency also began a program in which Americans were sent abroad to network with drug counselors, physicians, and governmental ministers in an effort to enlist all elements of the world population in the war against cocaine.

DEMOGRAPHICS

Cocaine use has plateaued in the United States. It is estimated that 10 percent of all Americans have tried cocaine at least once and 4 million Americans use cocaine on a regular or semi-regular basis. Approximately 5 to 7 percent of all adolescents, 25 to 30 percent of young adults and approximately 9 to 10 percent of all adults have at least experimented one time with cocaine. Approximately one-third of all college students and 17 percent of all high school seniors have used cocaine at least once.

Cocaine use is found in all social classes and all geographic areas of the United States. The greatest rate of cocaine addiction is found in the metropolitan areas. Crack tends to be used by lower socioeconomic groups and powder cocaine by higher socioeconomic groups.[13,14,15]

PHARMACOLOGY

Cocaine can be absorbed from all mucosal areas of the body. Most commonly, it enters via the nasal mucosa and the lungs. It can also be injected or smoked. Powder cocaine (cocaine hydrochloride) is a water soluble compound that can be absorbed from the serum after being dissolved in water and injected. It can also be directly absorbed through the nasal mucosa.

If cocaine hydrochloride is dissolved in a strong basic compound and the base is extracted by a solvent such as ether, a solid form of cocaine is obtained called crack. Crack becomes volatile at just under 100° C, so it is smoked. The smoked crack, however, is not absorbed through nasal mucosal but through the villi of the lungs.

Whereas intravenous cocaine produces an effect in one minute, smoking of free-base cocaine produces a high within only 10 seconds. Intranasal cocaine produces onset of action in 3 to 4 minutes with a duration of 30 to 45 minutes. Intravenous cocaine hydrochloride produces results within 30 to 45 seconds with a "high" of 20 minutes duration. Smoking cocaine produces a high within 8 to 10 seconds with a duration of 5 to 10 minutes.[16]

Cocaine is metabolized primarily in the liver. The major active metabolite is norcocaine, which is produced by N-demethylation. De-esterification produces two inactive metabolites, benzoylecgonine and ecgonine methyl ester. This latter metabolite is formed by both plasma choline esterase as well as hepatic cholinesterase.[17]

The major psychiatric activity of cocaine is produced by its action upon the neurotransmitter dopamine in the major pleasure center of the brain, the nucleus accumbens. By its activity in these areas, cocaine is able to supplant water as well as food and sex as primary drives. It then becomes *the* primary drive. As a primary drive, it can compel drug seeking behavior.

Cocaine acts on dopaminergic neurons, producing a massive release of dopamine into the synaptic cleft. Cocaine then blocks the re-uptake of dopamine, maintaining a high level of concentration at the postsynaptic receptors. Therefore, increased dopamine stimulation occurs on a short-lived basis producing primary drive/reward sensations in the ventral tegmentum as it projects to the striate, limbic and cortical dopamine areas.

Because much of the intrasynaptic dopamine is blocked from intraneuronal uptake, it cannot be broken down by intraneuronal monoamine oxidase (MAO) into homovanillic acid (HVA) and recycled. It is metabolized instead by interneuronal catechol-O-methyltransferase (COMT) into 5-hydroxytyramine, which cannot be recycled. Thus, with each cocaine-induced dopamine stimulation cycle, the dopamine supply is slowly but progressively depleted. According to this model, the rapidly occurring tolerance, craving and addiction is a function of progressive dopamine depletion.[18-21]

MEDICAL COMPLICATIONS

A variety of medical complications are produced by cocaine. Many of these are relatively minor and include nose bleeds, sinusitis, and rhinitis. Secondary but more serious affects include hepatitis and acquired immune deficiency syndrome, as well as sepsis, meningitis and endocarditis which arise from the use of infected needles.

Repeated nasal constriction caused by cocaine insufflation can cause necrosis of the mucosal tissue and eventually perforation of the cristae gallae. This can lead to the leakage of cerebral spinal fluid as well as disruption of the integrity of natural barriers to ingress into the brain.[22] Both meningitis and encephalitis can result.[23]

Cocaine appears to deregulate the TRH-TSH-thyroid axis.[24] Cocaine use also causes cardiovascular morbidity. Vascular complications include thrombosis, embolization, and hemorrhagic pseudotumors.[25]

The major cardiac complications include ischemia and arrythmia. Cocaine produces ischemia through coronary arterial spasm. Myocardial ischemia begins when the cardiac demand for arterial blood exceeds the supply. By potentiating the physiological response to catecholamines, cocaine elevates blood pressure increasing the myocardial oxygen-demand. However, cocaine also exerts a direct vasoconstrictor effect on smooth vascular muscle. In spite the increased demand for myocardial oxygen, this profound vasoconstriction may overwhelm auto-regulatory mechanisms which ordinarily preserve coronary blood flow, thus producing ischemia.[26-28]

Ischemia is a major element in producing myocardial infarction. A second element is cocaine-facilitated platelet aggregation, which produces coronary thrombosis. Cocaine potentiates these coagulant effects by transient depletion of protein C and antithrombin III. Cocaine patients are frequently found with myocarditis and dilated myocardiopathy probably due to hypersensitivity, catecholamine-induced focal myocarditis.

Cocaine may produce reentry tachycardia as well as ventricular arrhythmias. The arrhythmias may take the form of accelerated idioventricular rhythms, ventricular tachycardia, or ventricular fibrillation. These conditions, for the most part, however, occur in the presence of underlying cardiac pathology. Cocaine apparently produces pathological effects by blocking sodium channels. This blockage alters impulse conduction and results in conduction delays coupled with unidirectional blockade. This produces a reentry circuit for the tachyrhythmia.[29-30]

The cardiotoxic effects of cocaine can be intensified by the concurrent use of alcohol. A combination of cocaine and ethanol can result in the hepatic production of "cocaethylene." Unlike cocaine, this compound has low effect on serotonergic receptors. Since serotonin tends to depress dopamine activity, cocaethylene is thus able to produce a more intense dopaminergic effect on the brain and myocardium. In Dade County, Florida, the lethality of cocaethylene was demonstrated in a series of post mortem examinations. Of 237 cocaine-related deaths, 124 post-mortem serum samples were positive for the cocaine-ethanol combination and 77 for cocaethylene. It is estimated that 40 percent of all alcohol-cocaine abusers produce cocaethylene.[31-35]

The pregnant patient is at particular risk. Pregnant cocaine abusers have an increased rate of spontaneous abortion due to a abruptio placentae and placenta previa. Babies born to crack-abusing mothers manifest a particular syndrome and are called "crack babies." They tend to be jittery, floppy, and of small size, with congenital heart and skull defects. These defects are thought to be due to dose-dependent fetal hypoxemia, tachycardia, and hypertension.[36-40]

DIAGNOSIS

Acute use of cocaine in any form produces the characteristic and highly desirable rush. There is a feeling of euphoria with increased libido, increased energy, and indifference to cold, thirst and hunger. If the patient should overdose, usually by injection, a variety of symptoms may be manifested. These include arrhythmias, circulatory failure, convulsions, emesis, auditory and visual hallucinations, hyperreflexia, hypertension and muscle spasms with increased restlessness and tonic-clonic seizures.

During chronic abuse, the patient's mood progresses from grandiose and euphoric states to dysphoric ones. Affect, however, remains labile.[41] There also may be anxiety, auditory and visual hallucinations (usually of small darting objects), paranoia, progression of psychosis, and possible violent or irrational behavior. Chronic abusers also note formications (i.e., a sensation similar to ants crawling on or underneath one's skin).

Because of cocaine's chronic inhibitory effect of dopamine recycling and production, there is hypoprolactemia.[42] Other less common findings include dental carries due to decreased salivary secretion and the pain-masking effects of cocaine on the oral mucosa.

Due to anorexigenic effects of cocaine, there is generalized weight loss and malnutrition. The combination of carries and weight loss has sometimes been confused with bulimia. Malnutrition may sometimes be associated with deficiencies of thiamine, folic acid, vitamin B6 and vitamin C due to the anorexigenic effects of this drug.

Though acute cocaine use is associated with increased sexual performance, chronic use leads to sexual dysfunction and decreased libido. Addicts who chronically insufflate cocaine present with necrosis of the nasal septum and the crista galli. This results in loss of the sense of smell, sinusitis, epistaxis, and leakage of CSF into the nostrils. There may also be chronic pneumonia due to a diminished immune response.[43]

During withdrawal, the patient appears extremely dysphoric. Usually there are complaints of severe abdominal cramping. There is also constriction of the pupils, general hypotension and hyporeflexia. Penile erection and piloerection are often seen. Patients tend to have a ravenous appetite. This hyperphagia can also be accompanied by specific cravings for salty and/or fatty foods such as French fries or potato chips.[44]

The specific symptoms of withdrawal can often be superimposed upon symptoms of chronic abuse, which at times can make diagnosis difficult. However, in making a diagnosis, it is important to recognize the principles of the medical/biopsychiatric approach.

Acute cocaine use causes a massive release of catecholamine, centrally and peripherally. Therefore, there is a stimulation of the cerebral cortex, lower brain centers, and the cord reflexes. Patients tend to be "wired," i.e., there is hyperactivation of the brain and body. Chronic depletion of the catecholamines, dopamine, and norepinephrine as well as other monoamines, cause the patient to "run-down." There is a need for food, water, and rest. The muscles, which were hyperstimulated, go into spasms which manifest as abdominal cramping.[45]

see p 73

hypo

TREATMENT

Treatment of cocaine abuse is tripartite. It involves pharmacological detoxification; pharmacological and medical support including treatment of complications due to cocaine; and a supportive, integrated medical/psychiatric approach to the underlying causes of the addiction.

Detoxification is most often accomplished by using the bromocriptine-desipramine protocol regimen. Since cocaine withdrawal is due to depletion of dopamine, many researchers began experimenting with a number of dopamine agonists to counter withdrawal symptoms. Bromocriptine and amantadine are both used for this purpose.[46,47] Bromocriptine has generally produced more consistent results although there have been problems with nausea in some research paradigms.[48,49] Dopamine depletion and hyperprolactemia have been reported to be effectively normalized by bromocriptine.

While bromocriptine reduces the withdrawal symptoms, it does not affect the cocaine craving. Desipramine, a noradrenergic agonist, has been reported to chemically reverse this craving by producing beta-adrenergic and dopaminergic subsensitivity. A number of researchers have reported that desipramine produces relief from cocaine cravings within two to three weeks, the approximate time needed to induce receptor subsensitivity.[50,51] When combined (see Table 6-1), bromocriptine and desipramine can effectively reduce craving and other withdrawal effects of cocaine.[52] Although the table displays a 12-day withdrawal regimen, the protocol can be accelerated when the necessary dosages are titrated against side effects and symptoms.

Cardiovascular complications are a major hazard of cocaine addiction withdrawal. Severe hypertension caused by cocaine-induced α-adrenergic release can be treated by labetalol (Normodyne, Trandate) 2 mg. per minute administered as a continuous infusion. Beta-adrenergic blockers such as propranolol HCl (Inderal) can be useful to manage ventricular tachyarrhythmias or superventricular arrhythmias.

A controversial area is the use of thrombolytic agents to treat cocaine-induced myocardial infarction. In the case of myocardial ischemia or *impending* myocardial infarctions, however, it is generally accepted that prompt treatment with calcium channel blockers such as nifedipine (Procardia); 10 mg. by mouth sublingually can effectively reduce spasms.[53,54]

see p 203

Table 6-1: Recommended Bromocriptine-Desipramine Protocol for Cocaine Detoxification

Day	Bromocriptine Dosage	Desipramine Dosage
1	2.5 mg. four times daily	50 mg. at bedtime
2	2.5 mg. four times daily	50 mg. at bedtime
3	1.875 mg. four times daily	100 mg. at bedtime
4	1.875 mg. four times daily	100 mg. at bedtime
5	1.25 mg. four times daily	150 mg. at bedtime
6	1.25 mg. four times daily	150 mg. at bedtime
7	0.625 mg. four times daily	Continue 200 mg. at bedtime for 1 to 8 mos.
8	0.625 mg. four times daily	
9	0.625 mg. three times daily	
10	0.625 mg. three times daily	
11	0.625 mg. twice daily	
12	0.625 mg. twice daily	
13	0.625 mg. per day	
14	Discontinue	

The biopsychosocial aspects of cocaine addiction are dependent on several factors. These include the absence or presence of specific gateway drugs; underlying psychological factors such as the presence of a depression; and biological factors. Gateway drugs vary from locale and may determine the age at which the patient is introduced to cocaine. These gateways drugs may include alcohol, marijuana and volatile agents.

Psychologically, some cocaine addicts have an underlying depression or dysthymia and use cocaine as a form of self-medication. Other patients may be involved in a job or academic situation in which they are called upon to produce amounts of energy, creativity or dynamism which they feel they do not possess. They may temporarily find these attributes within themselves in the initial stages of cocaine addiction.

The genetic component may also determine if the patient shall be addicted to cocaine. Recently, researchers at the National Institute of Drug Abuse cloned a gene for the protein upon which cocaine acts to produce a characteristic rush. It may be, then, that the prolonged action of dopamine in the synaptic cleft is dependent upon the availability and action of this specific protein. This may point to a personal predilection for selective attraction to cocaine.

Detoxification is usually accomplished on an inpatient unit so that the patient may receive prompt attention for the more painful aspects of withdrawal. These include abdominal cramping and hallucinations as well as potentially dangerous cardiovascular complications and neurological complications of withdrawal. In therapy, a team approach is sought in which symptom reduction, medical monitoring, supportive psychotherapy, and investigation into the patient's environment and personality are carried on concurrently.

After detoxification, the patient can be discharged into the community with close monitoring.[55,56] Some clinicians prefer a day-center approach which provides therapy for only part of the day. When not in therapy, the patient goes to work or school and sleeps at home. In these partially integrated environments, the recovering abuser can resolve interpersonal problems on a continuing basis while also finding recreation and developing friendships within a peer-support network of recovering abusers. Former addicts are better able to maintain their new lifestyles. Cocaine Anonymous and Narcotics Anonymous can provide the fellowship which is a very necessary part of the recovering process.

A certain subpopulation of patients, however, are not able to enter society without continuous work- and home-support systems. Therefore they are involved in economically integrated, self-supporting, and in many cases self-sufficient communities. Here the recovering patient works, sleeps, eats and recreates within the psychological and geographical confines of his therapeutic drug community. Notable examples are the San Patrignano Foundation near Rimini, Italy, and DeLancey Street Foundation in San Francisco and New York City.[57,58]

TYPICAL CASE PRESENTATION

The patient is a 24-year-old white male who presented to his family doctor's office complaining of an itch that was driving him "crazy." In her notes, the physician recorded that the patient was "hyperactive, very edgy, speech was pressured and he kept moving around the room." In addition there was elevated blood pressure of 150/90, tachycardia of 89 beats/minute, and mydriasis. Closer examination revealed inflammation of the nasal mucosa with some "nasal drip." Deep tendon reflex was extremely brisk.

The doctor ordered a SMAC, CBC-Diff, urinalysis and a qualitative urine drug screen. When the laboratory reports revealed the presence of benzoylecgonine, she confronted the patient and recommended inpatient detoxification. The patient agreed to be detoxified on a medical unit.

After admission but prior to detoxification, the patient admitted to the staff that he had visual hallucinations of small darting objects. The staff members also noted paranoid persecutory delusions, pressured speech, tremors and mydriasis. A urine and serum drug screen done by GC/MS was positive for benzoylecgonine. The patient gave a history of insufflating "about $2,000 of coke a week." He denied use of alcohol or other drugs.

Therapy was initiated with bromocriptine 25 mg. four times a day, orally, and desipramine 50 mg. orally before sleep. Because of agitation and anxiety he was prescribed hydroxyzine 50 mg. every 6 hours or as needed, orally. The dosage of bromocriptine was gradually decreased over a two week period and discontinued on day 14. Desipramine was increased up to 3200 mg. before sleep by the eighth day and maintained.

During detoxification the patient began complaining of abdominal cramping with hyperphagia and a craving for salty foods. This was treated by doubling the size of his meal portions and giving him unlimited potato chips. Muscular cramping in the extremities was noted and treated with light massage.

After detoxification, the patient was placed in an outpatient rehabilitation center. Therapy focused on his feelings of being overwhelmed by his work schedule as a sales-director. He noted cocaine helped him "go all night." He also had recent troubles with potency and therefore feelings of inadequacy were addressed. Since he was involved with a drug abusing subculture and lover, steps were taken to remove him from his social environment. He received support from both Cocaine Anonymous and Narcotics Anonymous support groups which he attended 5 nights per week during active rehabilitation and three nights weekly post-discharge.

NOTES

1.   Giannini AJ, Loiselle, RH, Giannini MC. Space-based abstinence. Clin Toxicol, 1988; **25**:463.
2.   Siegel RK. Cocaine smoking. J Psychoactive Drugs 1982; **14**:271-359.

3.   Haas LF. Coca shrub (Erythroxylum coca). J Neurol Neurosurg Psychiatry 1995; **59(1)**:25.

4.   Stewart DJ, Inaba T, Lucassen M, et al. Cocaine metabolism: cocaine and norcocaine hydrolysing by liver and serum esterases. Clin Pharmacol 1979; **25**:464-468.

5.   Watson WA, Wilson BD, Roberts DK. Clinical interpretation of urine cocaine and metabolites in emergency department patients. Ann Pharmacother 1995; **29(1)**:82.

6.   Schiwy-Bochat KH, Bogusz M, Vega JA, Althoof H. Trends in occurrence of drugs of abuse in blood and urine of arrested drivers and drug traffickers in the border region of Aachen. Forensic Sci Int 1995; **71(1)**:330-42.

7.   Wang WL, Darwin WD, Cone EJ. Simultaneous assay of cocaine, heroin and metabolites in hair, plasma, saliva and urine by gas chromatography-mass spectrometry. J Chromatogr B Biomed Appl 1994; **660(2)**:279-90.

8.   Beltran R, Bell T, Fisher S, Ros S. Utility of laboratory screening in cocaine-exposed infants. Clin Pediatr 1994; **33(11)**:638-5.

9.   Bruns AD, Sieske LA, Jacobs AJ. Analysis of the cocaine metabolite in the urine of patients and physicians during clinical use. Otolaryngol Head Neck Surg 1994; **111(6)**:722-6.

10. DeGiovanni N, Strano Rossi S. Simultaneous detection of cocaine and heroin metabolites in urine by solid-phase extraction and gas chromatography-mass spectrometry. J Chromotogr B Biomed Appl 1994; **658(1)**:69-73.

11. Quinn T, Shannon E. Sweet, sweet surrender. Time 1994 (Nov 7); **145**:46-48.

12. The wages of crack. The Economist 1994; **134**:29-30.

13. MacDonald DI. High school senior drug use declines. JAMA 1987; **257**:2699.

14. Abelson HI, Miller JD. A decade of trends in cocaine use in the household populations. Natl Inst Drug Abuse Res Monogr Ser 1985; **61**:35-49.

15. Court C. Report paints picture of global use of cocaine. BMJ 1995; **310(6983)**:825-6.

16. Javaid JI, Musa MN, Fischman MW et al: Kinetics of cocaine in humans after intravenous and intranasal administration. Biopharm Drug Dispos 1983; **4**:9-18.

17. Faraj BA, Davis DC, Camp VM, Mooney AJ 3rd, Holloway T, Barika G. Platelet monoamine oxidase activity in alcoholics, alcoholics with drug dependence, and cocaine addicts. Alcohol Clin Exp Res 1994; **18(5)**:1114-20.
18. Dackis CA, Gold MS: New concepts in cocaine addiction: The dopamine depletion hypothesis Neurosci Biobehav Rev 1985; **9**:469-477.
19. Satel SL, Krystal JH, Delgado PL, Kosten TR, Charney DS. Tryptophan depletion and attenuation of cue-induced craving for cocaine. Am J Psychiatry 1995; **152(5)**:778-83.
20. Pulvirenti L, Koob GF. Dopamine receptor agonists, partial agonists and psychostimulant addiction. Trends Pharmacol Sci 1994; **15(10)**:374-9.
21. Spealman RD, Bergman J, Madras BK, Kamien JB, Mella KF. Role of D1 and D2 dopamine receptors in the behavioral effects of cocaine. Neurochem Int 1992; **29(March suppl)**:147S-152S.
22. Ashchi M, Wiedemann HP, James KB. Cardiac complication from use of cocaine and phenylephrine in nasal septoplasty. Arch Otolaryngol Head Neck Surg 1995; **121(6)**:681-4.
23. Reevey RR, McWilliams ME, Fitz-Gerald M. Cocaine-induced ischemic cerebral infarction mistaken for a psychiatric syndrome. South Med J 1995; **88(3)**:352-4.
24. Giannini AJ, Malone DA, Loiselle RH. Blunting of TSH response to TRH in chronic cocaine and phencyclidine abusers. J Clin Psychiatry. 1987; **48**:25-29.
25. Herning RI, Glover BJ, Koepple B, Phillips RL, London ED. Cocaine-induced increases in EEG alpha and beta activity: evidence for reduced cortical processing. Neuropsychopharmacology 1994; **11(1)**:1-9.
26. Kolodgie FD, Farb A, Virmani R. Pathobiological determinants of cocaine-associated cardiovascular syndromes. Hum Pathol 1995; **26(6)**:583-6.
27. Willens HJ, Chakko SC, Kessler KM. Cardiovascular manifestations of cocaine abuse. A case of recurrent dilated cardiomyopathy. Chest 1994; **106(2)**:594-600.
28. Rump AF, Theisohn M, Klaus W. The pathophysiology of cocaine cardiotoxicity. Forensic Sci Int 1995; **71(2)**:103-15.

29. Shen WK, Edwards WD, Hammill SC, Bailey KR, Ballard DJ, Gersh BJ. Sudden unexpected nontraumatic death in 54 young adults: a 30-year population-based study. Am J Cardiol 1995; **76(3)**:148-52.

30. Schindler CW, Tella SR, Erzouki HK, Goldberg SR. Pharmacological mechanisms in cocaine's cardiovascular effects. Drug Alcohol Depend 1995; **37(3)**:183-91.

31. Tardiff K, Marzuk PM, Leon AC, Hirsch CS, Stajic M, Portera L, Hartwell N. Cocaine, opiates, and ethanol in homicides in New York City: 1990 and 1991. J Forensic Sci 1995; **40(3)**:387-90.

32. Pirwitz, MJ, Willard JE, Landau C, Lange RA, Glamann DB, Kessler DJ, Foerster EH, Todd E, Hillis LD. Influence of cocaine, ethanol or their combination on epicardial coronary arterial dimensions in humans. Arch Intern Med 1995; **155(11)**:1186-91.

33. Higgins ST, Budney AJ, Bickel WK, Foerg FE, Badger GJ. Alcohol dependence and simultaneous cocaine and alcohol use in cocaine-dependent patients. J Addict Dis 1994; **13(4)**:169-76.

34. Bailey DN. Cocapropylene (propylococaine) formation by human liver in vitro. J Anal Toxicol 1995; **19(1)**:1-4.

35. Perez-Reyes M. Jeffcoat AR, Myers M, Sihler K, Cook CE. Comparison in humans of the potency and pharmacokinetics of intravenously injected cocaethylene and cocaine. Psychopharmacology 1994; **116(4)**:406-6.

36. Madden JD, Payne TE, Miller S. Maternal cocaine abuse and effect on the newborn. Pediatrics 1986; **77**:209-211.

37. Chasnoff IJ, Bussey ME, Savish R. Perinatal cerebral infarction and maternal cocaine use. J Pediatr 1986; **108**:456-459.

38. Hepper PG. Human fetal behavior and maternal cocaine use; a longitudinal study. Neurotoxicology 1995; **16(1)**:139-43.

39. Buehler BA. Cocaine: how dangerous is it during pregnancy? Nebr Med J 1995; **22(4)**:708-2.

40. Mirochnick M, Frank DA, Cabral H, Turner A, Zuckerman B. Relation between meconium concentration and the cocaine metabolite benzoylecgonine and fetal growth. J Pediatr 1995; **126(4)**:636-8.

41. Giannini AJ, DeFrance KT, Loiselle RH. Reception of nonverbal communication in alcoholics. J Gen Psychology 1984; **116**:241-244.

42. Dackis CA, Estroff TW, Gold MS. Hyperprolactinemia in cocaine abuse. Am Psych Assoc Abstr 1985; **NR**:181.

43. Daras M, Tuchman AJ, Koppel BS, Samkoff LM, Weitzner I, Marc J. Neurovascular complications of cocaine. Acta Neurol Scand 1994; **90(2)**:124-9.

44. Giannini AJ, Miller NS, Loiselle RH, Turner CE. Cocaine associated violence and route of administration. J Sub Abuse Treatment 1993; **10**:67-70.

45. Pugh CM, Mezghebe HM, Leffall LS, Jr. Spontaneous bowel perforation in drug abusers. Am J Emerg Med 1995; **13(1)**:113-5.

46. Tennant FS, Sagherian AA. Double-blind comparison of amantadine hydrochloride and bromocriptine mesylate for ambulatory withdrawal from cocaine dependence. Arch Inter Med 1987; **147**:109-112.

47. Giannini AJ, Sullivan BS, Loiselle RH. Comparison of bromocriptine and amantadine in the treatment of acute cocaine withdrawal. Soc Neurosci Abstr 1987; **13(1)**:88.

48. Dackis CA, Gold MS, Sweeney DR, et al. Single-dose bromocriptine reverses cocaine craving. Psychiatry Res 1987; **20**:261-264.

49. Giannini AJ, Baumgartel P, DiMarzio LR. Bromocriptine therapy in cocaine withdrawal. J Clin Pharmacol 1987; **27**:267-270.

50. Gawin FM, Kleber HD. Cocaine abuse treatment: Open pilot trial with desipramine and lithium carbonate. Arch Gen Psychiatry 1984; **11**:903-904.

51. Giannini AJ, Malone DH, Giannini MC, et al. Treatment of depression in chronic cocaine and phencyclidine abuse with desipramine. J Clin Pharmacol 1986; **26**:211-214.

52. Giannini AJ, Billet W. Bromocriptine-desipramine protocol in treatment of cocaine addiction. J Clin Pharmacol 1987; **27**:259-554.

53. Gioil G, Manuel M, Russell J, Heo J, Iskandrian AS. Myocardial perfusion pattern in patients with cocaine-induced chest pain. Am J Cardiol 1995; **75(5)**:396-8.

54. Bunn WH. Giannini AJ. Cardiovascular complications of cocaine abuse. Am Family Physician 1992; **46**:769-774.

55. Havassy BE, Wasserman DA, Hall SM. Social relationships and abstinence from cocaine in an American treatment sample. Addiction 1995; **90(5)**:699-710.

56. Hoffman JA, Caudill BD, Koman JJ 3rd, Luckey JW, Flynn PM, Hubbard RL. Comparative cocaine abuse treatment strategies: enhancing client retention and treatment exposure. J Addict Dis 1994; **13(4)**:115-28.

57. Festinger DS, Lamb RJ, Lountz MR, Kirby KC, Marlowe D. Pretreatment dropout as a function of treatment delay and client variables. Addict Behav 1995; **20(1)**:111-5.

58. AJ Giannini. Mi rintroni in mente. Il Giornale di San Patrignano. 1990; **6(32)**:27-28.

CHAPTER 7

KHAT

The khat bush is the single largest source of naturally occurring sympathomimetics in the world. With the exception of the cocoa leaf, its stimulant effects are more powerful than that of any other botanical. The khat plant itself is a thick bush which grows from 2 to 12 feet in height in the sandy soil of the Mideast. It is legal everywhere in the world with the singular exception of Uganda.

The khat plant (*Catha edulis*) has been used in Middle Eastern cultures in a similar manner as cocaine was used by the Incan culture in South America. When the freshly picked young leaves of the khat plant are chewed, a highly stimulant effect is produced. These effects are due to the large number of sympathomimetic phenylalkylamines: cathine (norpseudoephedrine), cathinone [(-)-α-aminopropiophenone], phenylpropanolamine, cathedulin (pentahydroxy-sesquiterpene) and cathidine (euoniminol).

Khat is used as a social drug in Yemen, where it replaces alcohol among devout Moslems. Khat is also used extensively in the horn of Africa. Its use in Djibouti has caused great economic distress and has led to a balance of payments problem due to decreased economic productivity. In addition to its recreational attraction, khat can be utilized to alleviate effects of fatigue, hunger and thirst.[1,2]

LABORATORY TESTING

Of the various constituents of khat, cathinone is the most important.[3] Cathinone can be tested by thin layer chromatography and gas chromatography. Thin layer chromatography can produce a number of false positives, and misidentification with amphetamines and cocaine is common. Also, khat leaves are a mixture of numerous constituents some of which are legal in the United States. These include phenylpropanolamine and norpseudoephedrine, found in many over-the-counter cold medications. Khat constituents can also be detected in the serum within 12 hours, and in the urine within 12 to 24 hours after chewing. Salivary testing produces positive results within a few seconds.[4,5]

HISTORY

The first historical reference to khat occurred in the campaigns of Alexander the Great. Alexander apparently sent khat to one of his generals, Harrar, to cure a depressive state which was interfering with his martial duties. In the 10th century, the Arabic physician Ahmid Al-Biruni recommended khat infusions as "a refrigerant for the stomach and liver." In 1237, a Yemeni physician, Naquib Al-Din Al-Samarqandi, prescribed khat for "treatment of melancholia."

Khat addiction was first documented in the case of an Ethiopian tribal chief, Amda Sion, who ruled the city of Marade the 14th century. Because of his addiction and the subsequent addiction of his court, he was easily defeated by an Arabic general, Sabra Al-Din. To keep his newly conquered population in subjugation, Sabra began planting khat throughout his conquered province. He did this to enervate his newly won subjects, much as Amda Sion inadvertently enervated his own army.

The first European to describe khat was the explorer Barthelem D'Herbelot DeMolainville in 1603. In 1775, it was classified botanically by a student of Linnaeus, Petrus Forskal. It has kept the initial classification, *Catha edulis*, to this day. Khat was then studied by a number of Europeans. In 1841, a Frenchman, Dr. Paul Bottan, definitively described the cultivation and clinical effects of khat including its addictive potential. Because of this addictive potential, khat use was popularized by the English explorer Sir Richard Burton in a series of articles and books in 1856. In 1861, samples of khat were imported to Europe by the French explorer Antoine Petite en Quartone Dillon.

The 20th century's attitude towards khat became increasingly negative. Investigating Italy's new African colonies, the Italian physicians Carlo Gennora and Giovanni Rovesti described khat as a folk medicine of ambiguous effect. The French physicians working on the indigenous tribes of Harrar concluded that khat was responsible for dementia and heart disease. These reports effectively aborted a nascent French industry in khat whereby khat infusions, khat elixirs, khat syrups and khat tinctures were used to treat various "maladies nerveuses de femme."

An English pharmacist, W. Martindale, manufactured various khat preparations including "catha cocoa milk" (a mixture of khat, milk and glycerol phosphate) as a "nerve tonic" and a mixture of khat and phenolphthalein for use as a mild laxative. Because of the Italian and French reports, however, khat use died out. This happened in spite of the granting of a Swiss patent for an extract of catha leaves.

Khat use was not observed again in the Western world until 1984, when researchers described khat-induced mania in the United Kingdom. Then, in 1993, a case of khat psychosis was found in the United States.

Since khat leaves must be chewed within three days of being picked, khat use is dependent on the smuggling of khat plants to the United States. These plants are then repotted and grown in situ. Due to relatively brief duration of a jet flight, freshly picked khat leaves can be flown to all parts of the European continent.

DEMOGRAPHICS

Khat abuse, when initially described, was limited to populations in the Mideast as well as Middle Eastern immigrants to the West. Generally it was abused within ethnic enclaves by resident and alien populations, as well as by Middle Eastern college students at American and European universities. Khat came to the attention of the Western public during the Gulf War and the subsequent Somali incursion of 1993. The popular press reported extensively on this drug and it became an element of street pharmacopoeia. Interestingly, soldiers who were exposed to khat in both these military campaigns appear not to have brought back the habit of khat chewing to their native countries.[6]

CHEMISTRY AND PHYSIOLOGY

Khat is not a pure compound but rather a complex mixture of a number of drugs, not all of which have sympathomimetic qualities. Therefore, khat chewing has effects not only upon catecholamines but upon beta-endorphins, thyroid hormone and testosterone.[7,8]

Habitual chewers of khat have increased urinary levels of all catecholamines but decreased levels of metabolites. This effect is thought to be due to an amphetamine-like inhibition of monoamine activity. Chronic and occasional khat users also have elevated levels of both serum ACTH and cortisol. Habitual use of khat produces elevated beta-endorphin levels and decreased prolactin levels; single dosing or occasional use produces an opposite effect.

While the effects of khat on ACTH, HGH, and prolactin are similar to those of amphetamine, its effects on beta-endorphin are not. Sympathomimetic effects of khat are similar to those seen with other sympathomimetics such as cocaine and amphetamine. These include hyperalertness, increased socialization, and hypersexuality followed by hyposexuality. A sense of well being at the initial phase of addiction is follow by irritability or depression. Clinical observations included elevated diastolic and systolic blood pressure, tachycardia, atrial and ventricular arrhythmia, mydriasis, flushing and tremors. In most subjects both rectal and axillary body temperatures are elevated.

Chronic khat use has been associated with anorexia, diminished libido, and an indifference to cold. Chronic use, however, produces no change in respiratory rate or heart rate. Sleep pattern, although initially unaffected, eventually is notable for insomnia, hypersomnia or a combination of these states. Formications have been observed in later stages of addiction.[9,10]

Animal studies have shown clonus, stereotypy, and hypothermia in both rats and mice. Isolated mouse hearts treated with khat extract display both increased dynotropic and chronotropic activity. Isolated sections from a variety of animal sources treated with cathinone displayed smooth muscle relaxation with a subsequent decrease in parastolic contraction frequency and contraction intensity.

In addition to its effect on beta-endorphin, cathinone has other opioid effects. Its use as an analgesic has been documented for at least 200 years. In the mouse, cathinone increased the latency during the hot plate test and inhibited response to intraperitoneal administration of acetic acid. Both the acetic acid test and the hot plate test responses where inhibited only by α-methyltyrosine, α-methyl-P-tyrosine, and diethylcarbamate, as well as naloxone.[11-14]

There is also some evidence that khat acutely affects the posterior pituitary gland. Nearly half of khat chewers experience polyuria, thirst and dryness. Approximately one-third of all chewers note dysuria, fever and fatigue after periods of prolonged chewing.

The major psychoactive constituent of khat is cathinone [(-)-α-propiophenone], a phenylalkylamine. Cathinone exists in three forms. It is, however, highly unstable and decomposes rapidly, giving rise to a large number of decomposition (not metabolic) products. Many of these decomposition products are also psychoactive.

Cathinone is also a biosynthetic intermediate of ephedrine which is also a psychoactive constituent of khat. A related product is (-)-norephedrine.

A unique phenylalkylamine found in the khat leaf is cinnamoylethylalmine, which is chemically similar to cinnamedryl, an ingredient of over-the-counter preparations for menstrual cramping. Other important phenylalkylamines are phenylpropanolamine and cathedulin (pentahydroxy-sesquiterpene) series. Cathedulin exists in approximately 19 forms in the khat plant.

Several major flavonol glycosides are present in khat: kempferol, quercetine, myristicine and 3-O-rhamnoside. These flavonols may produce hallucinogenic experiences. A number of other volatile compounds including numerous terpinoids and aromatic compounds have been isolated but their psychoactive activity has not yet been established.[4,6,7]

Rat and mouse studies as well as human studies suggest that cathinone has an amphetamine-like releasing effect on catecholamine storage sites. Cathinone apparently blocks presynaptic intraneuronal dopamine re-uptake and subsequent metabolism by intraneuronal monoamine oxidase (See Chapter 3, Amphetamines). Khat seems to affect the limbic system, locus ceruleus, pars compactum, nucleus circumbins, cingulum gyrus, infundibulum, and possibly the pontine raphi nuclei. Acutely, cathinone enhances the release of biogenic amines. Its peripheral effects include myogenic, especially cardiac and gastrointestinal activity. These appear to be due to direct release of transmitters from catecholamine storage sites such as the adrenal gland. Analgesia and anesthesia seem to be due to opiate mechanism plus a nonopiate mechanism which involves a spinal reflex.[15,16]

DIAGNOSIS

Khat intoxication differs from khat addiction, yet both are similar to that seen in other sympathomimetics.[17] Chewing of khat causes an immediate rise in blood pressure which peaks within three hours and slowly returns to normal after sixteen hours of discontinuance of chewing. Heart rate peaks within 90 minutes returning to normal within three to four hours. There is a rise in body temperature of approximately 1°C within 90 minutes of ingestion. This continues for several hours thereafter and then decreases so that an overall minor loss of body temperature of an additional 0.5°C is seen after 16 hours. Respiratory rate tends to increase by approximately 6 respirations per minute.[8]

The average subject's rate rises from 21 to 28 respirations per minute after three hours, but then falls to approximately 19 respirations per minute after 16 hours. The heart rate increases to approximately 15 beats per minute after 90 minutes slowing to 7 or 8 beats per minute. After 16 hours, this tachycardia reverses itself and ends. This tachycardia is not associated with electrocardiographic changes, however.[18]

Reaction time is reduced from 3.5 seconds to 2.6 seconds after 90 minutes, and to 2.5 seconds after three hours. After 16 hours, there is an increased reaction time of 3.8 seconds. Deep tendon reflexes tend to increase by 70 percent in all abusers immediately after chewing khat leaves. There is also a noticeably dry mouth and an urge to urinate. After three hours post chewing, there tends to be a feeling of fatigue and exhaustion associated with perspiration. There is difficulty urinating but sexual desire is increased. Most users report a marked loss of appetite and at least one-third reported transient constipation.

Long term abuse tends to be associated with anxiety and confusion. The patient tends either to be very extremely dysphoric or aggressive and agitated, especially if he has been denied access to his source. Because of inhibition of thirst, the khat patient tends to be emaciated and dehydrated. Visual hallucinations and paranoia have been described in single case studies. Tachycardia is common and some nonspecific arrhythmias have been occasionally reported. There are fine to coarse resting tremors and occasional tics or twitches. While some patients may be anxious or depressed, others may be excited, euphoric or grandiose. Flushing is noted but most often in the acute stage.[19,20]

Electroencephalograms have demonstrated some increase in slow-wave activity. Formications and mydriasis have been noted in some chronic abusers. Changes in sleep patterns include insomnia, hypersomnia, or any consistent combination of these two. There is a gradual tolerance to heat and cold.[21]

TREATMENT

Pharmacological treatment of acute khat intoxication is generally not necessary. If the patient seems to be agitated and on the verge of loosing self-control, hydroxyzine HCl 50 mg. intramuscularly, or lorazepam

2 mg. intramuscularly, given once or twice over a four hour period is usually adequate. Chronic depression responds best to noradrenergic antidepressants such as amitriptyline HCl or fluoxetine at daily dosages of 200 to 250 mg. and 50 to 100 mg., respectively. When withdrawal symptoms are very uncomfortable and the patient has used large amounts of the drug (i.e, more than 20 leaves per day over 8 or more months), the patient can be detoxified with bromocriptine as per the chart in Chapter 6, Cocaine.[22,23]

TYPICAL CASE PRESENTATION

The patient is a 28-year-old recent immigrant from a Middle Eastern country. He has chewed khat throughout his adult life. After coming to the United States, he brought with him several fresh cuttings of khat which he planted in numerous pots throughout his home. For the past two years in this country, he was able to cultivate and chew khat on a daily basis. In the past 8 months, due to the impending breakup of his marriage, he began chewing larger amounts of khat on a near-continuous basis. Recognizing his problem, he presented to the emergency room.

The patient presented with flushed skin, gross resting and physiological tremors, and a mild to moderate intention tremor. Pupils were moderately dilated, speech was pressured, and associations were flighty. Vital signs included tachycardia with a heart rate of 94 beats per minute and blood pressure of 160/110 mm/Hg. Respirations were approximately 30 per minute. At this point, the patient admitted he had chewed a mouthful of khat while driving to the hospital emergency room. Bowel sounds were decreased but sphincter tone was increased. Laboratory testing was negative for all compounds studied including phenylpropanolamine.

The patient was then admitted and detoxified with bromocriptine 0.625 mg. four times a day on a tapering basis for four days. After this time the bromocriptine was discontinued and he was sent to an outpatient drug rehabilitation program. While in the program, he developed depression which was successfully treated with Prozac 20 mg. every day over a two-month period.

NOTES

1. Giannini AJ, Burge H, Price WA, Shaheen JA. Khat: another drug of abuse? J Psychoactive Drugs 1986; **18**:155.
2. Kalix P Khat: a plant with amphetamine effects. J Substance Abuse Treat 1990; **5**:163-169.
3. Kalix P. The amphetamine-like releasing effect of the alkaloid cathinone on rat nucleus. Neuropsychopharmacol Biol Psychiatr 1982; **6**:43-49.
4. Manciuli M, Parrinello A: Il gat (*Catha edulis*). La Clinica Therapeutica 1967; **43**:103-172.
5. Pantelis C, Hindler CG, Taylor JC. Use and abuse of khat (*Catha edulis*): a review of the distribution, pharmacology, side effects and a description of psychosis attributed to khat chewing. Psychol Med 1989; **19(3)**:657-658.
6. Ahmad AM, Anania MC, Nencini P. Long lasting analgesic effects of cathinone. Proceedings of the International Conference on Khat, Antananaurivu, Madagascar, 1983.
7. Widler P, Mathys K, Brenneisen R, Kalix P, Fisch HU. Pharmacodynamics and pharmacokinetics of khat: a controlled study. Clin Pharmacol Ther 1994; **55(5)**:556-562.
8. Zelger JL, Schorno HX, Carlini EA. Behavioral effects of cathinone, an amine obtained from *Catha edulis* Forsk: comparisons with amphetamine, norpseudoenphedrine, apomorphine and nomifensine. Bull Narc 1980; **32(3)**:67-81.
9. Schechter MD, Rosecrans JA, Glennon RA. Comparison of behavioral effects of cathinone, amphetamine and apomorphine. Pharmacol Biochem Behav 1984; **20(2)**:181-184.
10. Heymann TD, Bhupulan A; Zureikat NE, Bomanji J, Drinkwater C, Giles P, Murray-Lyon IM. Khat chewing delays gastric emptying of a semi-solid meal. Aliment Pharmacol Ther 1995; **9(1)**:81-3.
11. Nielsen JA: Cathinone affects dopamine and 5-hydroxy-tryptamine neurons in vivo as measured by changes in metabolites and synthesis in four forebrain regions in the rat. Neuropharmacology 1985; **24(9)**:845-852.
12. Tariq M, Parmar NS, Qureshi S, el-Feraly FS, Al-Meshal IA. Clastogenic evaluation of cathinone and amphetamine in somatic cells of mice. Mutat Res 1987; **190(2)**:153-157.

13. Huang D, Wilson MC. The effects of dl-cathinone, d-amphetamine and cocaine on avoidance responding in rats and their interactions with haloperidol and methysergide. Pharmacol Biochem Behav 1984; **20(5)**:721-729.

14. Schechter MD. Rats become acutely tolerant to cathine after amphetamine or cathinone administration. Psychopharmacology 1990; **101(1)**:126-131.

15. Kalix P. Hypertensive response to cathinone, an alkaloid of *Catha edulis* (khat). J Pharm Pharmacol 1980; **32**:662-664.

16. Kalix P. Hypermortality of the amphetamine type induced by a constituent of khat leaves. Br J Pharmacol 1990; **68(1)**:11-13.

17. Giannini AJ, Castellani SA. A manic like psychosis due to khat. J Toxicol: Clin Toxicol 1982; **19**:455-454.

18. Kalix P. Cathinone, a natural amphetamine. Pharmacol Toxicol 1992; **70(2)**:77-86.

19. Mack RB. Khat on a hot tin roof. *Catha edulis* intoxication. N C Med J 1995; **56(2)**:112-4.

20. Jager AD, Sireling L. Natural history of khat psychosis. Aust N Z J Psychiatry 1994; **28(2)**:331-2.

21. Kalix P. Khat, an amphetamine-like stimulant. J Psychoactive Drugs 1994; **26(1)**:69-74.

22. Giannini AJ, Martin DM, Turner CE. Treatment of khat addiction. J Substance Abuse Treat 1992; **9**:379-382.

23. Giannini AJ, Nakoneczie AN. Treatment of khat addiction with bromocriptine mesylate. Am J Therapeutics 1995; **2**:487-489.

CHAPTER 8

MARIJUANA

see p 97

Of the psychoactive substances available in the Americas, Europe and Japan, marijuana is the drug most often abused. Its psychoactive effects are a function of 400 potential psychoactive ingredients found in the marijuana plant itself, as well as a function of other drugs which are used to accentuate the drug's effects. It can be smoked alone or mixed with a variety of compounds including phencyclidine, crack cocaine, formaldehyde and lime.[1] It can be brewed as an infusion and sometimes mixed with chocolate, catnip, or chamomile. It is sometimes chewed with ashes or betel nut. Marijuana is often soaked in solvents, including formaldehyde, kerosine and some insecticides. Marijuana is also baked in a variety of pastries.

In popular parlance, marijuana is the dried plant, *Cannabis sativa*, which is smoked. Hashish is the resin of the marijuana plant and hashish oil is the refined resin.

LABORATORY TESTING

Laboratory testing for marijuana can include testing of several hundreds of psychoactive substances. Practically however, most clinical testing is for Δ-9-tetrahydrocannabinol (THC).

Of the marijuana which is smoked in cigarette form, 20 to 80 percent of the resultant THC reaches the lungs but only an average of 15 to 17 percent of this becomes bioavailable. The THC is rapidly metabolized into many forms, therefore peak blood levels are generally low, in the 30 to 50 ng. per ml. range. The half-life of the drug is 56 hours in occasional users but only half of that in chronic users. Because THC is lipid soluble, it can be detected up to 120 hours after last use.[2,3]

Testing is usually done for the major metabolites. Although THC can be detected in the feces and with difficulty in the serum, urinary samples are preferred. Generally, enzyme multiplied immunoassay (EMIT) and radioimmunoassay (RIA) are used for screening tests. Gas chromatography (GC) in combination of mass spectrometry (MS) is used to confirm positive results, especially in legal proceedings. Thin-layer chromatography (TLC) is used in some legal jurisdictions. It is a screening test which is not very sensitive and generally gives an unacceptable amount of false negative results. Sensitivity of RIA for THC is approximately 2 to 10 ng. per ml. and for EMIT 20 to 100 ng. per ml. The reliability of EMIT is 97 to 99 percent; that of RIA is approximately 97 percent. With all types of tests mentioned including TLC, false negatives tend to be more common than false positives.[4,5]

HISTORY

The first medical notation of marijuana was documented in the *Herbals* of the Chinese emperor, Chen Nung, 1000 years B.C. Egyptian historians of the pharaonic Middle Kingdom included in their chronicles the self-destruction of the Scythian empire due to enervation of its soldiers by marijuana. There also appear to be two separate notations of marijuana in the Old Testament of the Bible. The Israelite King Solomon mentions marijuana approvingly in his "Song of Songs." In the later book of Tobias, the eponymous protagonist finds a grieving widow. He discovers that her previous seven husbands had died of asphyxiation on their wedding night because of the presence of a marijuana brazier in her wedding chamber. He disposes of the problem by marrying the wealthy widow and neutralizing the effects of marijuana with fish entrails and ashes.[6]

In classical literature, Homer's *Iliad* records the gift of marijuana from Helen to Telemachus. Greek oracles would burn laurel or marijuana leaves in a brazier and inhale their smoke before uttering their prophetic announcements. The physician, Galen, noted its use in the treatment of otitis media in the Roman Empire. *The Thousand and One Nights* of Haroun Al-Rashid recorded its use by Scheherazade in her seduction of the caliph.

In the thirteenth century, the Persian warlord and mystic Naguib Ad-Din was able to recruit large numbers of soldiers for his small mercenary army by intoxicating them with hashish and then spiriting them from their villages. Under the influence of hashish, his troops were waited upon by female courtesans and plied with delicacies. After they awoke from their hashish-intoxicated night of pleasure, they were told they had been to Paradise and would return again during their martyrdom. Having once "died and gone to heaven," these troops fought willingly and ably as "assassins" (users of hashish).

As hashish use became more popular, Arabic rulers began to mobilize against the enervation of their populations. The first official move was made by the Emir Soundouni She'houni in the Arabian Peninsula. In 1378, he prohibited the use of hashish and punished anyone who used or cultivated the plant by forcibly extracting their teeth. This move was not at all effective. The Arabian historian Al-Magrizi later ascribed the general decline of Egyptian society to hashish abuse.[7]

Marijuana was introduced to the Western hemisphere in the early 1500's. African slaves brought marijuana plants with them to the Portuguese colony of Brazil, while the Spaniards began growing it in Chile. The Spaniards initially used it as a source of industrial fiber while the Brazilians used it as a medicine and intoxicant. From the Americas it was reintroduced to Europe. In 1735, Linnaeus assigned it to the name *Cannabis sativa.*[8]

Cannabis was introduced to the Virginia colony of Jamestown in 1611 and later to the Massachusetts Bay colony in 1629. Although it was used primarily as a source of fiber, it was sometimes smoked. It became a source of medicinals and was grown by many American planters, including George Washington and Thomas Jefferson.

By the mid-eighteenth century, tincture of marijuana was produced commercially in Philadelphia by John Biddle. Its use was endorsed by Dr. Benjamin Rush, the founder of the American Psychiatric Association. In 1839, Dr. William O'Shaughnessy recorded the use of cannabis as an analgesic, anticonvulsant and muscle relaxant in Calcutta, India. Upon returning from India, he popularized its use in medical circles. As a result, leading physicians such as the notable Sir William Osler recommended it for migraine headaches. By 1850, it was listed in the *U.S. Pharmacopoeia*, and it was manufactured by a number of leading pharmaceutical houses including Burroughs-Wellcome, Eli Lilly and Parke-Davis.

Widespread recreational abuse of marijuana also began at that time. The nineteenth century psychopharmacologist, Jacques Joseph Moreau, in his experiments with marijuana, ate hashish and became intoxicated by it. He introduced the practice of eating hashish to Alexander Dumas and Charles-Pierre Baudelaire with whom he formed "Le Club Des Haschischins" in Paris. An American writer, Fitz-Hugh Ludlow, popularized his experiences with the book, *The Hasheesh Eater.*

Cannabis was legally but surreptitiously smoked in "hashish houses." Marijuana reached into mainstream American society as a result of American military incursions into Central America and the Caribbean. As the soldiers returned from their assignments, they brought back the ritual of "smoking reefer." During the 1920's, it was enjoyed with bathtub gin and the other speakeasy delights. With the repeal of Prohibition, Harry Anslinger, director of the Federal Bureau of Narcotics, focused the efforts of the Bureau towards the criminalization of marijuana use. As a result of his efforts, the Marijuana Tax Act of 1937 drastically curtailed marijuana abuse.

In the 1950's, the "beat" generation adopted marijuana as a result of use by its poets and writers, and as a rebellion against Eisenhower "normalcy." Marijuana later became part of the antiwar protest movement.

As a result of pressures by social activists and ad hoc marijuana lobbying organizations such as NORML (National Organization for the Reform of Marijuana Laws), marijuana was potentially decriminalized in the Comprehensive Drug Abuse Prevention and Control Act of 1970. As a result of this act, the penalties for marijuana use became substantially less than those for other drugs such as cocaine or heroin. Marijuana was further decriminalized by Alaska and Oregon, where marijuana ranks as a minor misdemeanor in Oregon and has been recriminalized in Alaska.

Marijuana use has generated some minor literary productions. In Lewis Carrolls' *Alice in Wonderland* and later *Through the Looking Glass*, John Tenniel, an illustrator, included numerous renderings of the marijuana plant. The 1930's film *Reefer Madness* is now seen as a campy B-movie propaganda piece espousing the negative effects of marijuana use. The "beat" poetry of Allen Ginsberg and Laurence Ferlingehetti and the prose of John Kerouac, which describe the effects of marijuana, are still read today.

DEMOGRAPHICS

Marijuana has become an indigenous, subsistence cash crop in exporting nations. Some individual Europeans, North and South Americans grow their own marijuana, and it is also an export crop from Latin America. The country of origin determines the form of marijuana exported: the dried marijuana plant is often exported from Latin American countries, the Caribbean and Southeast Asia; hashish and hash oil usually come from the Middle East, Turkey, Azerbaijan, Georgia,

Armenia, and North Africa. Currently, 20 million Americans smoke marijuana at least once per month. Of these, nearly half admit to smoking it once a week and 6 million on a daily basis.

Marijuana abusers are sometimes polydrug abusers. Five percent of those who use marijuana on a daily basis use it with alcohol, 7 percent with crack cocaine, 1 percent with phencyclidine and 2 percent with other illicit drugs. There is also a specific subgroup that mixes marijuana with formaldehyde, strychnine, stramonium, catnip and asthmador.[9]

The typical abuser is a man or woman in his or her late 20's. Users are most often introduced to marijuana in junior high or middle-school. They are generally employed in a low-skilled occupation and can live in an urban, suburban or rural area. There is a high amount of absenteeism at work and school. They are usually not academically or vocationally ambitious. After three years of chronic use, sexual activity becomes low and the social circle tends to be limited to other marijuana abusers. Abusers usually rationalize their declining performance and life situation. They generally have minor legal problems including DUI convictions, minor theft, and "disturbing the peace" citations.[10]

PHARMACOLOGY

Although marijuana is a widely used drug, its effects are poorly understood. Marijuana includes several different classes and contains nearly 400 different chemical forms. There are also at least 200 psychoactive substances in marijuana. Of these substances, 64 are cannabinoids. However, only 14 of these cannabinoids have been studied.

It is generally agreed that the most psychoactive cannabinoid is a form of THC, though it is not known whether Δ-9-THC or its active metabolite 11-OH-Δ-9-THC is the source of major effects. The route of ingress of THC determines speed of onset. The effects of smoked marijuana may persist for 12 to 24 hours. These effects are less intense and of longer duration than ingested marijuana.

Intravenous administration brings about rapid although inconsistent effects. Absorption of smoked marijuana occurs approximately within 7 to 10 minutes with a steady decline over three hours. Ingestion of marijuana produces onset of effects within one-half to two hours, although this can vary according to type of food or gastric contents. Use of hashish or hash oil does not increase peak absorption or intensity of effects.[11]

see p 23

After intake, the active metabolite Δ-9-THC is partially bound to albumin. It then undergoes a biphasis metabolism. It is transformed into the inactive metabolite 8-11-DiOH-THC and the highly active metabolite 11-OH-Δ-9-THC. This latter active compound is then converted into another metabolite which is inactive.

Generally, the first half-life has a duration of one to four hours. The second half-life lasts approximately 30 hours and represents mobilization of 11-OH-Δ-9-THC from lipid storage depots as well as similar storage sites in muscle tissue.

Thirty to sixty percent of THC in all its forms is excreted through the feces. The remaining amount is excreted in the urine. Most of the inactive metabolites of 11-OH-Δ-9-THC are excreted exclusively in the urine while 11-OH-THC and 11-OH-Δ-9-THC are excreted both in the urine and feces. The trace amounts of Δ-9-THC are excreted in equal proportions in the urine and feces. Because of the very high lipid solubility of marijuana as compared to other drugs of abuse, 25 percent of marijuana intake is excreted during the first seven days post-usage.

Not much is known of the action of marijuana because most of its hypothesized activity is based upon empirical evidence or association. Because of its sedating effects, many authors have inferred activation of the benzodiazepine (B-Z) receptors in the limbic system and cerebellum. Others have viewed the same activity as evidence of glutamate receptor activity while a third group has conjectured the existence of a specific THC receptor. Because of its effects on REM sleep, it is thought that marijuana also acts on a serotonin receptor site.[12]

The impairment of memory, especially memory storage, suggests activity in the hippocampus and implies dopamine activity. The effect on aggressivity implies both serotonin and dopamine activity. Because marijuana is a drug with addictive potential, many researchers have inferred drive-state activity in the primary pleasure centers of the brain. It thus may act upon the nucleus accumbens through mesolimbic pathways and the pars compacta, including the frontal cortex through mesocortical pathways. Activity at these sites may enhance drug-seeking behavior by reinforcing activity in the ventral tegmentum through post-synaptic neurons.[13,14]

Marijuana also apparently acts on cholinergic systems. The brain contains a memory and storage amplification system called the "Papez circuit." This circuit acts to intensify memories with an emotional matrix. Memories which are transferred from the hippocampus through the hypothalamic mamillary bodies to the anterior thalamus receive emotional enforcement. From the anterior thalamus, fibers are sent to the cingulate gyrus, then projected to the retrosplenial cortex and finally descending back to the hippocampus. In this manner a closed reverberating circuit is achieved by which new memories are processed for storage and invested with an emotional overlay.

Marijuana amplifies the pleasurable memories associated with intoxication and disrupts other memories to create a self-perpetuating positive reinforcement system. Marijuana's effect on the reward system of the primary pleasure pathways are dopaminergic. The memory-emotional amplification coinvolves cholinergic activity.[14]

A phenomenon seen in marijuana addiction is that of post reverse tolerance. In most addicting drugs, tolerance is achieved so that increasingly higher doses are needed to stabilize withdrawal symptoms and give the pleasurable effect. In a few studies, marijuana abusers seemingly needed progressively lesser amounts as the addiction progressed. This reverse-tolerance, however, is a pseudophenomenon due to the storage of the highly lipophilic Δ-9-THC and its metabolites in fat and muscle tissue. The lipid saturation of the stored drug is a phenomenon almost unique to marijuana. The release of stored marijuana into the blood supply accounts for this pseudophenomenon.[15]

DIAGNOSIS

Acute effects of marijuana include multiple visual distortions such as the singular phenomenon of inanimate objects seeming to "breathe" (i.e., having small but definite contractions and expansions). There is also diminished attention span and concentration, impaired balance with Romberg's sign, depersonalization, derealization, orthostatic hypotension, drowsiness sometimes paradoxically associated with hyperalterness, tachycardia, diminished coordination, increased reaction time, and diminished deep tendon reflexes. When the marijuana is smoked, there is usually conjunctival injection.

Chronic use is associated with an "amotivational syndrome." This syndrome is a triad of antisocial behavior, apathy and disinterest. These are accompanied by diminished drive and ambition, diminished motivation, poor judgement, distractibility and social avoidance. There is also fragmentation of thought and decline in habits, hygiene and communication.[16]

The suspiciousness seen in chronic use may progress to paranoid persecutory delusions reinforced by auditory and visual hallucinations. There is also depression, which is usually but not always partially alleviated by continued use of marijuana. This is associated with a high potential for suicide and accompanied by feelings of helplessness, hopelessness, lethargy, anergia, anhedonia, tearfulness, and a sense of anomie. Anxiety may occur independently or accompany the depression. There is diminished appetite and diminished libido. Men in particular have decreased sexual performance. In addition to the decreased libido there is partial impotence and ejaculatory inhibition.[17,18]

Chronic use of marijuana has multiple medical effects. Studies have suggested but not proven diminished pulmonary macrophage activity. Other studies have implied a decreased lymphocyte genesis. This apparently improves after cessation of marijuana use. Another temporary effect is diminished levels of luteinizing hormone, which can increase the number of anovulatory cycles in females. In males, there is a decrease in follicle stimulating hormone, a decrease in testosterone production, possible atrophy of the testicles, and pseudobreast formation.[19,20] While chronic marijuana can elevate carboxyhemoglobin levels and exert a negative inotropic effect, these actions have only limited clinical significance unless the subject has severe cardiac impairment.

Some gastric distress is dose-related in chronic marijuana users. Clinical symptoms include emesis, diarrhea and increased frequency of bowel movements. This is due to changes in the gastrointestinal system that increase gastric emptying time and decrease gastrointestinal motility.

No neurological effects have been proven to be associated with marijuana though some clinicians have described marijuana-induced seizures.[21]

Smoking marijuana is associated with chronic bronchitis, chronic cough, respiratory depression, and increased incidence of pneumonia. There are also decreased forced expiratory volume and decreased diffusing capacity. There are also case reports, but no study, of marijuana pulmonary hypertension syndrome.[22]

TREATMENT

Acute detoxification of marijuana is seldom necessary in adults. When there is agitation, hydroxyzine 50 mg. intramuscularly is effective. Some clinicians have recommended 2 grams of caffeine benzoate intramuscularly to enhance metabolism, although the utility of this treatment has not been necessarily proven. Acute psychosis can be treated with haloperidol 5 mg. intramuscularly.

The only reliable recorded case of marijuana overdose occurs in the pediatric literature. If a small child should have access to marijuana in any form, emesis should be induced by magnesium sulfate or syrup of ipecac if ingestion has occurred. Respiration should be supported and blood pressure should be maintained with norepinephrine (Levophed) 2 ampules per 250 cc to 500 cc of 0.4 saline, titrating the solution against the blood pressure.

Chronic treatment includes use of phenothiazines or butyrophenones for paranoid delusions or hallucinations. Marijuana-induced depression appears responsive to either noradrenergic, serotonergic, or dopaminergic antidepressants. The choice should be dependent upon the clinician's experience and patient response. Generally, antidepressant doses have been administered at the higher range.

Because of the use of adulterants with marijuana, their presence should be ascertained by laboratory testing. If such a presence is noted, their pathological effects upon the patient should be treated adjunctively with the marijuana addiction treatment. In addition to drug screening, laboratory testing should include a minimum of a CBC-Diff and an SMA-18 to ascertain liver or kidney damage. Because of the effects of marijuana upon an unborn child, pregnancy tests should be ordered. Babies whose mothers have used cannabis during the pregnancy generally have increased startle response and tremors. Long-term effects have not been adequately described.

TYPICAL CASE PRESENTATION

The patient was an 18-year-old high school student who was sent to a psychiatrist by her family doctor for treatment of depression. Her father gave a history of declining academic performance. He said that she had isolated herself from friends and family, spending many hours alone in a wooded lot near the home. The father, whose income was modest, was very concerned that her behavioral change would preclude a college scholarship. He further noted that she had quit the cheerleading squad and the school newspaper staff.

The patient was seen alone. She admitted to dysphoria lasting throughout the day. This was accompanied by anergia, anhedonia, and diminished concentration. She denied sleep difficulties. She said she had gained 4 pounds on a 5' 3" frame over six months and was concerned about this. She denied symptoms of anorexia and bulimia but did complain of loose stools. There was no history of laxative abuse.

The patient presented as a distracted young, white female in no acute distress. She appeared to have difficulty concentrating but was able to answer all questions appropriately. Because of the presence of an obvious hacking cough, she was questioned as to her smoking habits. She denied use of cigarettes or other tobacco products. When the psychiatrist persisted, she added "I said I don't smoke, unless you count marijuana." She then admitted to smoking up to five marijuana cigarettes per day.

During a family session, it was revealed that the patient began using marijuana "because my boyfriend asked me to." Her continuance was a result of poor family life occasioned by a mother who had a number of poorly-concealed extramarital affairs. Consequently, the patient found it necessary to overachieve to please her disappointed and lonely father. The father and daughter, but not the mother, agreed to enter family therapy. The daughter also received dyadic psychotherapy and fluoxetine 20 mg. every day for treatment of her depression. She also agreed to try Narcotics Anonymous.

NOTES

1. Hawkins KA, Schwartz-Thompson J, Kahane AI. Abuse of formaldehyde-laced marijuana may cause dysmnesia. J Neuropsychiatry Clin Neurosci 1994; 6(1):67.
2. Armbruster DA, Schwarzhoff RH, Pierce BL, Hubster EC. Method comparison of EMIT II and online with RIA for drug screening. J Forensic Sci 1993; 38(6):1326-41.
3. Bogusz M. Concerning blood cannabinoids and the effect of residual THCCOOH on calculated exposure time. J Anal Toxicol 1993; 17(5):313-6.
4. Cone EJ, Huestis MA. Relating blood concentrations of tetrahydrocannabinol and metabolites to pharmacologic effects and time of marijuana usage. Ther Drug Monit 1993; 15(6):527-32.
5. Starr K, Renneker M. A cytolic evaluation of sputum in marijuana smokers. J Fam Pract 1994; 39(4):359-63.
6. Balabanova S, Parsche F, Prisig W. First identification of drugs in Egyptian mummies. Naturwissenschaften 1992; 78(8):358.

7. Parsche F, Balabanova S, Pirsig W. Drugs in ancient population. Lancet 1993; **341(8843)**:503.

8. Prioreschi P, Babin D. Ancient use of cannabis. Nature 1993; **364(6439)**:186-7.

9. Hardert RA, Dowd TJ. Alcohol and marijuana use among high school and college students in Phoenix, Arizona: a test of Kandel's socialization theory. Int J Addict 1994; **29(7)**:887-912.

10. Yu J, Williford WR. The age of alcohol onset and alcohol, cigarette, and marijuana use patterns: an analysis of drug use progression of young adults. Int J Addic 1992; **27(11)**:1313-23.

11. Rinaldi L. Marijuana: a research overview. Alaska Med 1994; **36(2)**:107-13.

12. Iverson LL. Pharmacology. Medical uses of marijuana? Nature 1993; **365(6441)**:12-3.

13. Lundqvist T. Specific thought patterns in chronic cannabis smokers observed during treatment. Life Sci 1995; **56(23-24)**:2145-50.

14. Musty RE, Reggio P, Consroe P. A review of recent advances in cannabinoid research and the 1994 International Symposium on Cannabis and the Cannabinoids. Life Sci 1995; **56(23-23)**:1933-40.

15. Musty RE, Kaback L. Relationship between motivation and depression in chronic marijuana users. Life Sci 1995; **56(23-23)**:2151-8.

16. Solowij N. Grenyer BF, Chesher G, Lewis J. Biopsychosocial changes associated with cessation of cannabis use: a single case study of acute and chronic cognitive effects, withdrawal and treatment. Life Sci 1995; **5:56(23-24)**:2127-34.

17. Block RI, Ghoneim MM. Effects of chronic marijuana use on human cognition. Psychopharmacology (Berl) 1993; **111(2)**:163-8.

18. Chait LD, Perry JL. Acute and residual effects of alcohol and marijuana, alone and in combination on mood and performance. J Clin Pharmacol 1994; **115(3)**:340-9.

19. Dardick KR. Holiday gynecomastia related to marijuana? Ann Intern Med 1993; **119(3)**:253.

20. Thompson ST. Preventable causes of male infertility. World J Urol 1993; **11(2)**:111-9.

21. Brust JC, Ng SK: Hauser AW, Susser M. Marijuana use and the risk of new onset seizures. Trans Am Clin Climatol Assoc 1992; **103**:176-81.

22. Caiaffa WT, Vlahov D, Graham NM, Astemborski J, Solomon L, Nelson DE, Muñoz A. Drug smoking, pneumocystis carinii pneumonia, and immunosuppression increase risk of bacterial pneumonia in human immunodeficiency virus-seropositive injection drug users. Am J Respir Crit Care Med 1994; **150(6 pt 1)**:1493-1498.

CHAPTER 9

OPIATES

The opiates constitute a class of drugs that have been ambivalently regarded in both medicine, specifically, and in society, in general. This is due to the potential for addiction and social pathology inherent in this class of drugs that are the standard for the alleviation of major pain. Opiates can be either natural or synthetic. Natural opiates are derived from the sap of the poppy, *Papavera somnifera*. The sap contains raw opium which can then be further refined to produce morphine and then heroin. Semi-synthetic opiates include codeine and oxycodone. Meperidine, a totally synthetic drug, has a chemical structure only somewhat similar to opium but mimics much of its action. Methadone and propoxyphene, a methadone analog, do not share the chemical structure of opium but conformationally fit into the same receptor sites as the opiates. Unlike barbiturates, opiates have a valid, necessary use in medicine which is not duplicated by any other drug. As an analgesic, the opiates are widely available.

In the United States, multiple forms of opiates are available by prescription and heroin is widely available on the street. Thus, addicts have many options. They can obtain opiates legitimately from physicians or by stealing blank prescription forms, etc. They may get them from a relative or friend who has a documented need for such a drug and a valid prescription. They can also buy heroin from street dealers, although most street heroin is "cut" or diluted many times before it is sold to the addict. Generally, a 100 mg. bag of street heroin contains only 4 mg. to 10 mg. of the drug. It has become such that the true dosage of heroin is only a fraction of the stated dosage. However, sometimes stronger preparations will be sold and addicts overdose and die because they underestimate the strength. This is reportedly the reason for the death of the Sixties era rock singers Janis Joplin and Cass Elliott.

Table 9-1: Legal Opiates Available in the United States

Brand Name	Generic Name	Route of Administration
Alfenta	Fentanyl	I.M.
Anexsia	Hydrocodone	p.o.
Astramorph	Morphine	I.M.
Buprenex	Buprenorphine	I.M.
Dalgan	Dezocine	I.M.
Demerol	Meperidine	I.M., p.o.
Dilaudid	Hydromorphone	I.M., p.o., suppository
Duragesic	Fentanyl	Transdermal
Duramorph	Morphine	I.M.
Fentanyl	Fentanyl	I.M.
Hydrocet	Hydrocodone	p.o.
Hycodan	Hydrocodone	p.o.
Hydrostat	Hydromorphone	I.M.
Infumorph	Morphine	Epidural infusion
Innovar	Fentanyl	I.M.
Levo-Dromoran	Levorphanol	I.M., p.o.
Lorcet	Hydrocodone	p.o.
Lortab	Hydrocodone	p.o.
Mepergan	Meperidine; promethazine	I.M.
Metopon	Methydihydromorphone	I.M.
Nubain	Nalbuphine	I.M.
Numorphan	Oxymorphone	I.M. suppository
Oramorph	Morphine	p.o.
Percocet	Oxycodone	p.o.
Phocoldine	Pholdine	p.o.
Rescudose	Morphine	p.o.
Revia	Naltrexone	p.o.
Roxanol	Morphine	p.o.
Roxicodone	Oxycodone	p.o.
Sublimaze	Fentanyl	I.M.
Sufenta	Sufentanil	I.M.
Talacen	Pentazocine	I.M.
Talwin	Pentazocine, naloxone	I.M., p.o.
Tylenol II	Codeine	p.o.
Tylox	Oxycodone	p.o.
Trexan	Naltrexone	p.o.
Vicodin	Hydrocodone	p.o.

LABORATORY TESTING

All opiates can be tested by serum or urine samples. Because of the relatively short half-life, urine samples are preferred. Qualitative analysis is performed by thin layer chromatography. If conformation tests are required, gas chromatography/mass spectrometry (GC/MS) is preferred, though enzyme immunoassay (EMI) can also be used.[1]

GC/MS is preferred for a number of reasons.[2] First, it is more sensitive. EMI can detect down to 300 ng. per ml. while GC/MS has sensitivity of 200 ng. per ml. Second, GC/MS is more sensitive for ruling out false positives. Since poppy seeds have trace amounts of opium and codeine, a person eating a poppy seed pastry will test "positive" for opiates on nearly all tests. GC/MS identifies heroin abusers by the presence of the heroin metabolite, 6-monoacetylmorphine. Codeine and opium can be differentiated from a poppy seed confection by relative concentration. Using GC/MS, opiates can be tested up to 48 hours after last use.[3-6] (See Table 9-1.)

HISTORY

Opium use is thought to have originated in the Fertile Crescent of Iraq between the Tigris and the Euphrates rivers, during the Sumerian hegemony. From here, it was spread throughout the Middle East by their conquerors, the Akkadians under Sargon the First. The first documented evidence of opium use occurs in the third century B.C. manuscript of Theophrastus, a Greek philosopher and naturalist. Opium was then used intermittently throughout the classical world of Greece and Rome.

During the European Dark Ages (A.D. 476 to 1000), knowledge of opium disappeared from the monasteries of the scholarly monks. It was reintroduced to the European warrior class during the Crusades (1000-1300). At that same time, traders introduced it to China and India where it has been grown ever since. It was also during the Middle Ages that Paracelsus, a Swiss-born physician, prepared the first tincture of opium. Opium became popular in this form in eighteenth century Europe and much of Asia.

In the nineteenth century, opium use became fashionable and popular in Europe. The poet Elizabeth Barrett Browning was known for her afternoon teas made of infusions of roasted poppy seeds. Another poet, Samuel Taylor Coleridge, was addicted to laudanum (a mixture of alcohol, opiates and saffron) and reportedly produced some of his greatest poems, including the "Rime of the Ancient Mariner" and "Xanadu," under its influence. Thomas De Quincey's nineteenth century bestseller, *The Confessions of an English Opium Eater*, described for an enthralled Europe the torments of opium hallucinations and addiction. In America, opium dens were introduced to the United States by Chinese workers on railroads and in mining towns. The Civil War produced a generation of veterans who were addicted to tinctures of opium well into the twentieth century. Great Britain, in her imperial ventures with China, fought one of the first modern wars over drug addiction, the Opium War, in order to indirectly force the Chinese to buy and consume opium.

During the Victorian era, much research was done on opium. The chemist Serturner isolated the active ingredient of opium and named it "morphine" after the classical god of dreams, Morpheus. Within 25 years, Rogiquet, a French scientist, isolated codeine; and by 1850, the German physician Merck had extracted papaverine. In the 1850's, Bayer Laboratories had refined opium and patented a drug which was given the copyrighted name "Heroin." This was marketed as a nonaddicting analgesic. As a result, when Heroin's addicting nature became apparent, it was taken off the market and the copyright was withdrawn.[7]

Today, much of the heroin imported into the United States comes from the mountainous frontier provinces of Myanmar (formerly Burma) in southeastern Asia, although there are many other sources, including Mexico, Afghanistan, Pakistan and Turkey. It is estimated that 70 percent of all heroin entering the United States comes from the "Golden Triangle" — the area where the borders of Myanmar, Thailand and Laos meet.[7]

After the opium is processed into heroin, it moves across Europe, usually passing through Albania, Serbia or Austria. Albanian and Turkish gangs are estimated to control 70 percent of this distribution business. Albania also provides a depot for much of the heroin shipped to England and the Eastern Coast of the U.S.[8] Sixty percent of the heroin imported through America's East Coast is shipped from the ethnic Albanian village of Aveliki Trnovac in Serbia. The remaining 40 percent comes through village-based Nigerian gangs, though the Nigerian Drug Law Enforcement Agency under Maj. Gen. Musa Bamaiyi has somewhat reduced this trade. West Coast heroin is often imported by Chinese and Vietnamese gangs. Once received, heroin distribution is conducted by organized crime syndicates or gangs.[9]

DEMOGRAPHICS

The use of cocaine has seemingly legitimized opiates, giving a new cachet to many of its derivatives. Heroin snorting is now practiced by middle- and upper-class clientele who had previously scorned heroin as a "low-class drug."

There has also been a return to nineteenth century opium potions among boutique abusers. In 1992, there were reports from Oregon and Washington of the use of "opium tea," a powerful and addictive infusion. Laudanum is another retrograde form of opium which has been adopted by white upper-middle-class populations on the East and West Coasts. These forms of opium are addicting and quite illegal though they have been imbued with a nostalgic and legitimizing aura.[10,11]

The prevalence of heroin addiction in the U.S. is estimated at 2 percent. Most heroin addicts continue to utilize injectable heroin: this "traditional addict" accounts for 98 percent of all heroin abusers. Most use intravenous injection, although a minority might inject intramuscularly or insufflate. The typical abuser is an inner-city male who is single or divorced. He is usually poly-addicted, with alcohol being the most common collateral addiction.[12]

Twenty-five percent of all addicts die within 20 years of initial usage. The most common causes of death, in order of occurrence, are tuberculosis, hepatitis, suicide, homicide, AIDS, and trauma.[13,14]

In addition to the "boutique" and "traditional" opiate addict, there is the "medical" addict. Classically, this is a white male or female patient with a chronic or subchronic pain syndrome. As tolerance to the drug develops and the pain is unrelieved, the patient gradually passes from milder analgesics, such as propoxyphene, to pentazocine or oxycodone, to meperidine or hydromorphone, and finally to morphine injection. If cooperative or naive physicians are not available to write the desired prescription, the medical addict will forge or steal prescription pads or buy legitimate opiates "on the street."[15]

PHARMACOLOGY

The opiates of abuse are either opioid agonists or mixed opioid agonists/antagonists which work at all opioid receptors within the brain, whether the receptors are of the enkephalin, endorphin, or dynorphine subtype. Because mixed agonist antagonists such as pentazocine may displace heroin at endorphin receptor sites, a heroin addict who acutely switches to pentazocine may precipitate his own withdrawal.[16] Although nearly pure opiate antagonists exist, such as naloxone, they have no attraction to the addict and therefore no street value.[17,18]

Opiate receptors are distributed throughout the brain and spinal cord.[19] Those opiates that are distributed within the spinal cord, thalamus, and periaqueductal grey area mediate analgesia. Euphoria seems to be derived from various opiate actions upon the nucleus accumbens and, to a lesser degree, the ventral tegmental area in the mesolimbic system of the medial forebrain bundle and the limbic system. Withdrawal seems to be mediated by the periaqueductal grey area and the locus coeruleus.[20,21]

Within the locus coeruleus, opioid receptors are co-localized within α-2 receptors.[22] Activation of either of these receptors by opiate or α-2 agents produce adenylate cyclase inhibition. This then blocks the cyclic-AMP mediated opening of the potassium channels shared by both opiate and α-2 receptors. When opioid receptors are chronically stimulated with long term inhibition of adenylate cyclase, there were is a fall in the c-AMP levels. This produces active dephosphorylation of the receptors that maintain the potassium channels in the open state. Desensitization may be modulated by Ca-calmodulin dependent protein kinase.[23]

Opiates also act on the reticular activating system in the brain stem to diminish the formation of new memories and to cause sedation. These also act on the medullary chemotrigger, producing nausea and emesis. Opiate-induced peristalsis causes anorexia, emesis, constipation and obstipation.[24,25] Actions at other opioid receptor sites cause diminished release of cortisol, luteinizing hormone, and testosterone. While opiates may reduce immune responsivity, there is evidence that the immune system produces opiate antibodies.[26]

DIAGNOSIS

The intoxicated opiate addict presents generally in a euphoric state. The pupils tend to be constricted and deep tendon reflexes are decreased. He may be confused and disoriented. Visual hallucinations are rare. There tends to be flushing of the skin. Respiratory rate, heart rate and blood pressure are generally decreased. Content at times may be euphoric verging on paranoid grandiose. Although most patients are temperature insensitive, some patient complain of chills.

Patients who have injected heroin, especially from nonsterile and shared needles, may present with abscesses, track lines, skin ulceration, muscle fibrosis, and muscle necrosis. The risk of AIDS and hepatitis also accompanies shared needles. Injections of large amounts of opiates can produce wide pupillary dilation and respiratory distress.

The withdrawal state is associated with abdominal cramping, confusion, depression, and arthralgia. Cramping may progress to emesis or be associated with diarrhea. There is marked diaphoresis associated with hot and cold flushes and myalgia. There is a marked penile erection as well as pilomotor erection. The patient may complain of nausea but craves sweets. There may be twitching or tics progressing to true fasciculations. There will be elevation of heart rate, respiratory rate, and blood pressure.

The patient overdosing on opiates will generally be severely confused or comatose. There will be severe hypotension with respiratory depression which can proceed to respiratory arrest. There will be bradycardia and diminished bowel sounds. As a result of the respiratory depression, there will be hypoxia sometimes progressing to respiratory acidosis. There is generally a fever in excess of 100°F.

Outpatient therapy is difficult. This group of abusers often has highly developed manipulative skills.[27] The easy availability of opiates makes them susceptible to high levels of relapse. For those addicts using opiates to treat pain, the clinician must ascertain whether the pain is a self-reinforcing mechanism to obtain opiates. By reducing the source of pain, the opiate-seeking behavior may be reduced.[28] Medical interventions must be accompanied by individual and group supportive therapies. Because of cross sensitivity, the patient must be free from all addicting drugs, especially alcohol. Narcotics Anonymous should be an important support mechanism.[29]

TREATMENT

Pharmacological treatment of opiate addiction is divided into an acute and maintenance phases.

Acute chronic withdrawal can be treated with clonidine or methadone. Clonidine has several advantages: it is not a scheduled drug; it has absolutely no street value; and it produces rapid detoxification. Clonidine acts upon the α-2 receptors described above to inhibit the opiate-induced dephosphorization of the potassium channels. The withdrawal symptoms, which are a result of this phosphorylation, are greatly attenuated.

Clonidine is usually prescribed at a dosage of 17 μg. per kg. every day. This generally works out to approximately 0.1 mg. to 0.2 mg. every six hours orally. The dosage is gradually titrated downward over a four to five day interval.[30] In the special case of methadone withdrawal, maximum withdrawal symptoms occur after seven to fourteen days and the clonidine protocol should be used for a two or three week period.[31,32]

Methadone can also be used to treat opiate withdrawal. However, methadone itself is highly addictive and has value on the street. Generally, a test dose of methadone of approximately 10 mg. is given at the initiation of the detoxification protocol. After withdrawal symptoms appear, the same dose is increased until the patient is stable. The total dosage necessary to maintain stability in the initial 24-hour period is maintained for an additional 48 hours on a daily basis. The dosage is then decreased by 10 percent daily over the next 7 to 14 days. Unfortunately, many addicts cannot tolerate methadone withdrawal because of prolonged withdrawal symptoms.[33]

Methadone, however, is attractive as a maintenance drug for recovering opiate addicts. It is a long-acting agent which blocks the pharmacological effects of heroin. It also provides many of the attractive street effects of heroin. This is ambivalently viewed as a blessing. Methadone, however, maintains the intoxicated state including the effects of sedation. It also produces additive synergistic effects with alcohol.[34] (See Table 9-2.)

Naltrexone, which is also used in the treatment of alcohol addiction, blocks opiate activity at the endorphin receptor sites so that the opiate high is extinguished. The effects of naltrexone last approximately 24 hours, so it must be taken on a daily basis. Typically, naltrexone is given in the morning by a clinic because it is believed that a recovering heroin addict's ambition is at its highest in the morning.

While most patients present for detoxification, occasionally some may overdose. The initial treatment of overdose should be naloxone 0.4 mg. to 0.8 mg. by intravenous bolus every 20 minutes as necessary. If this dosage fails to reverse symptoms, increase naloxone dosage by 2 to 4 mg. increments until a maximum of 24 mg. per bolus is reached. Hypotension is treated conservatively by running 0.6 N saline intravenously, titrating the rate of drip against blood pressure. If this is not immediately successful, add phentolamine, two ampules per 250 cc of IV fluid.

Respiratory depression is sometimes associated with pulmonary edema. For respiratory depression, it is necessary to establish an artificial airway and maintain a total volume of 10 to 15 cc per kg. Generally, however, respiratory depression reverses with naloxone treatment. For pulmonary edema, ventilatory support and an oxygen line should be provided. In addition, furosemide 40 mg. should be given intramuscularly and repeated as necessary. An aminophylline rectal suppository is also indicated. Administer 40 to 60 percent oxygen via nasal catheter and utilize positive pressure breathing with surfactant if necessary. Three rotating tourniquets should be applied and changed every 15 minutes.

Table 9-2: Methadone and Methadone Derivatives Available in the United States

Brand Name	Generic Name	Route of Administration
Darvocet	Propoxyphene	p.o.
Darvon	Propoxyphene	p.o.
Dolophine	Methadone	p.o.
Methadone Diskets	Methadone	p.o.
PC-Cap	Propoxyphene	p.o.
PP-Cap	Propoxyphene	p.o.
Wygesic	Propoxyphene	p.o.

TYPICAL CASE PRESENTATION

A 29-year-old female presented at the emergency room in a comatose state. She was left by her boyfriend who then fled the scene. The patient's vital signs revealed blood pressure of 80/40 mm. Hg, a rectal temperature of 101°F, and a pulse rate of 55 beats per minute. Pupils were constricted and bowel sounds were decreased. Stat emergency room blood testing revealed the presence of respiratory acidosis. Examination of the extremities revealed multiple abscesses. Tracks followed the veins of the arms, and there was some woody induration present.

It was determined that the patient was in respiratory acidosis. Naloxone 0.5 mg. was given by intravenous bolus without result. The bolus was increased to 2 mg. and the patient became conscious but drowsy. This bolus was repeated over a six-hour period and the patient improved. She was then transferred from the emergency room to an inpatient detoxification service.

The patient was placed on clonidine 0.1 mg. every 6 hours and the dosage was gradually decreased by 20 percent decrements over a five-day period. During the detoxification period, the patient reported a craving for sweets, moderate abdominal cramping, and a craving for heroin. She was sent to an outpatient drug rehabilitation center for 6 weeks and placed on naltrexone 25 mg. every day with dosage to be monitored by the center.

NOTES

1. Joseph R, Dickerson S, Willis R, Frankenfield D, Cone EJ, Smith DR. Interference by nonsteroidal anti-inflammatory drugs in EMIT and TDx assays for drugs of abuse. J Anal Toxicol 1995; **19(1)**:13-7.

2. Colbert DL. Drug abuse screening with immunoassays: unexpected cross-reactivities and pitfalls. Br J Biomed Sci 1994; **51(2)**:136-46.

3. Hailer M, Glienke Y, Schwab IM, von Meyer L. Modification and evaluation of Abuscreen OnLine assays for drug metabolites in urine performed on a COBAS FARA II in comparison with EMIT d.a.u. Cannabinoid 20. J Anal Toxicol 1995; **19(2)**:99-103.

4. McCutcheon Jr, Wood PG. Snack crackers yield opiate-positive urine. Clin Chem 1995; **41(5)**:769-70.

5. Wasels R, Belleville F. Gas chromatographic-mass spectrometric procedures used for the identification and determination of morphine, codeine and 6-monoacetylmorphine. J Chromotogra A 1994; **675(1-2)**:225-34.

6. Abelson JL. Urine drug testing—watch what you eat! JAMA 1991; **266(22)**:3130-1.

7. Witkin G, Griffins J. The new opium wars. U.S. News and World Report 1994; **118(18)**:39-44.

8. The Albanian Connection. The Economist. 1994; **334**:61.

9. Nigerian drugs: internal trade. The Economist 1995; **336**:39

10. Hamilton K, Rossi M, Gegax TT. Back to Xanadu via Seattle. Newsweek 1994; **(Aug 29)**:62.

11. Wright JD, Pearl L. Knowledge and experience of young people regarding drug misuse, 1969-1994. BMJ 1995; **310(6971)**:20-4.

12. Jensen CF, Cowley DS, Walker RD. Drug preferences of alcoholic polydrug abusers with and without panic. J Clin Psychiatry 1990; **51(5)**:189-91.

13. Preston KL, Jasinski DR. Abuse liability studies of opioid agonist-antagonists in humans. Drug Alcohol Depend 1991; **28(1)**:49-82.

14. Blansfield HN. The care of injection-drug users with HIV infection. N Engl J Med 1994; **331(26)**:1774.

15. Bingle GJ, O'Connor TP; Evans WO; Detamore S. The effect of "detailing" on physicians' prescribing behavior for postsurgical narcotic analgesic. Pain 1991; **45(2)**:171-3.

16. Inciardi JA, Chambers CD. Patterns of pentazocine abuse and addiction. NY State Med J 1981; **71**:1727-1730.

17. Kolb VM. Opiate receptors: search for new drugs. Prog Drug Res 1994; **36**:49-70.

18. Rapaka RS, Porreca F. Development of delta opioid peptides as nonaddicting analgesics. Pharm Res 1991; **8(1)**:1-8.

19. Sabbe MB, Yaksh TL. The psychotomimetic effects of opiates and the sigma receptor. Neuropsychopharmacology 1990; **5(3)**:191-203.

20. Collin E, Casselin F. Neurobiological mechanisms of opioid tolerance and dependence. Clin Neuropharmacol 1991; **14(6)**:465-88.

21. Christie MJ. Mechanisms of opioid actions on neurons of the locus coeruleus. Prog Brain Res 1991; **88**:197-205.

22. Nistico G; Nappi G. Locus coeruleus, an integrative station involved in the control of several vital functions. Funct Neurol 1993; **8(1)**:5-25.

23. Mestek A, Hurley JH, Bye LS, Campell AD, Chen Y, Tian M, Liu J, Schulman H, Yu L. The human mu opioid receptor: modulation of functional desensitization by calcium/calmodulin-dependent protein kinase and protein kinase C. J Neurosci 1995; **15(3 Pt 2)**:2396-406.

24. Katzman MA, Greenberg A, Marcus ID. Bulimia in opiate-addicted women; developmental cousin and relapse factor. J Subst Abuse Treat 1991; **8(3)**:107-12.

25. Canty SL. Constipation as a side effect of opioids. Oncol Nurs Forum 1994; **21(4)**:739-45.

26. Loh HH, Smith AP, Lee NM. Effects of opioids on proliferation of mature and immature immune cells. Adv Exp Med Biol 1993; **335**:29-33.

27. Giannini AJ, Jones BT. Decreased reception of nonverbal cues in heroin addicts. J Psychology 1995; **119**:455-459.

28. Cherry DA, Gourlay GK. Pharmacological management of chronic pain: a clinicians perspective. Agents Actions 1994; **42(3-4)**:173-4.

29. Bhargava HN. Diversity of agents that modify opioid tolerance, physical dependence, abstinence syndrome, and self-administrative behavior. Pharmacol Rev 1994; **46(3)**:293-324.

30. Gold MS, Pottash ALC, Sweeney DR, Kleber HD. Opiate withdrawal using clonidine. JAMA 1980; **243**:343-344.

31. Gossop M, Battersby M, Strang J. Self-detoxification by opiate addicts. A preliminary investigation. Br J Psychiatry 1991; **159**:208-12

32. Trujillo KA, Akil H. Opiate tolerance and dependence: recent findings and synthesis. New Biol 1991; **3(10)**:915-23.

33. Reilly PM, Sees KL, Shopshire MS, Hall SM, Delucchi KL, Tusel DJ, Banys P, Clark HW, Piotrowski NA. Self-efficacy and illicit opioids use in a 180-day methadone detoxification treatment. J Consult Clin Psychol 1995; **63(1)**:158-62.

34. Kreek MJ. Biological correlates of methadone maintenance pharmacotherapy. Ann Med Interne (Paris) 1994; **145(Suppl 3)**:9-14.

CHAPTER 10

PHENCYCLIDINE AND THE DISSOCIATIVES

Phencyclidine (PCP) is the prototypical member of the "dissociatives," an entirely synthetic class of drugs (see Figure 10-1). PCP acts at multiple receptor sites and occurs in many active forms. It has been reported to have dopaminergic, serotonergic, noradrenergic, atropinic and opioid activity. Additionally, it has been manufactured and sold in volatile, liquid, powdered and crystalline forms. It can be injected, snorted, smoked, ingested or taken as an enema-preparation or douche.[1]

Because of its low price, multiple sites of action, and multiple physical forms, PCP can partially mimic other, usually more expensive, street drugs. In fact, 75 percent of all PCP sold is vended as another drug. Powdered PCP has been sold as amphetamine, methamphetamine, cocaine and paradoxically heroin and methaqualone, resulting in an odd mixture of stimulating and sedating effects. Liquid PCP or dissolved powdered PCP has been saturated into gels, paper and sugar cubes and then vended as LSD. It has been mixed with low-potency marijuana or bleached oregano and sold as high-THC content marijuana. Its tranquilizing and hallucinogenic actions plus its combustibility allow a PCP-oregano mix to be presented as high-quality marijuana.[2]

PCP can produce a constellation of symptoms including hypersexuality, hyperaggressivity, and anorexia, mimicking sympathomimetics such as amphetamine and cocaine. Its mixture of tranquilizing and anesthetic effects are similar to those of heroin or fentanyl, a narcotic analgesic. These same tranquilizing effects allow it to be unknowingly purchased in pill form as methaqualone or pentobarbital. Its hallucinogenic actions can be mistaken for those of LSD or DMT. On occasion, it has been saturated into different ornamental cacti which are then vended as "peyote," or into mushrooms which are presented as psilocybin.[2]

Figure 10-1: The Dissociatives

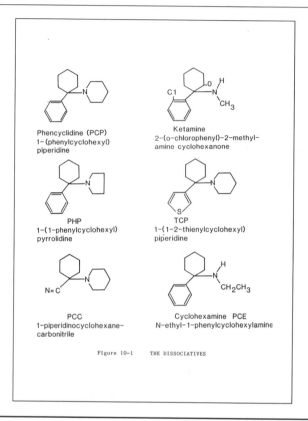

Phencyclidine (PCP)
1-(phenylcyclohexyl)
piperidine

Ketamine
2-(o-chlorophenyl)-2-methyl-
amine cyclohexanone

PHP
1-(1-phenylcyclohexyl)
pyrrolidine

TCP
1-(1-2-thienylcyclohexyl)
piperidine

PCC
1-piperidinocyclohexane-
carbonitrile

Cyclohexamine PCE
N-ethyl-1-phenylcyclohexylamine

Figure 10-1   THE DISSOCIATIVES

LABORATORY TESTING

The dissociatives PCP and ketamine can be detected by thin layer chromatography (TLC). However, PHP, a metabolite of PCP, cannot be detected by this method.[3]

While TLC cannot analyze many dissociatives, it seldom produces false positives. False positives can be reduced, however, and detection levels of all dissociatives including PHP can be increased by utilizing gas liquid chromatography (GLC), though it can produce false negatives when small amounts are tested. In cases when accuracy is absolutely necessary and cost is not a consideration, gas chromatography/mass spectrometry (GCMS) is preferred. Because the dissociatives act at a number of receptor sites, enzyme immunoassay (EIA) and radioimmunoassay (RIA) are not recommended due to the cross reactivity of these drugs and their metabolites with reagent antibodies.[4,5,6]

Since PCP is often vended as other, more expensive street drugs or is used as an adulterant in these drugs, it is recommended that a PCP analysis be included in all urine drug-screens.[7]

HISTORY

Phencyclidine, the first dissociative, was synthesized by Parke-Davis Laboratories in the 1950s. It was marketed under the trade name "Sernyl" as an anesthetic providing a smooth recovery without hang-over effects. In fact, the name Sernyl was chosen for the serene effects produced by this drug. This was based on the basis of animal studies which demonstrated that PCP was both a nonaddicting tranquilizer as well as a nonaddicting anesthetic that did not produce respiratory depression.

These animal studies, however, were unable to predict its effect in humans. The drug produced agitation, dysphoria, hallucinations, delirium and rage. In many cases, postoperative patients awoke in recovery rooms in the throes of frightening hallucinations, gripped by paranoid psychoses. Occasionally they became violent, injuring both themselves and the hospital staff. On one occasion, a patient undergoing a surgical procedure reached up and placed a strangling grip on the throat of the hovering anesthesiologist. As a result, Sernyl was withdrawn from the market in 1965.

In 1967, however, Parke-Davis reintroduced this product. It was sold as a veterinary anesthetic and tranquilizer under the name "Sernylan." Its reintroduction, unfortunately, was associated with the emergence of the drug culture in America.[8]

Phencyclidine was first reported as a drug of abuse in the Haight-Ashbury district of San Francisco in late 1967. Here it received its first street name, "the peace pill." Sernylan was much sought after because of its relatively low price, its nonaddicting "high," and the absence of specific federal or state laws prohibiting its use in humans. Its use spread quickly due to word of mouth throughout the West Coast. Because of publicity in the underground press, publications such as *Drum*, and sensational coverage in *Time*, Sernylan abuse spread nationwide.

Increased demand led to the manufacture of phencyclidine in underground laboratories. Relatively cheap raw materials such as piperidines and various ketones could be used to manufacture high-grade

PCP. Originally, nickel powder or US 5¢ coins were used as a catalyst with only moderately good results. Ironically, the introduction of automotive pollution control devices made platinum, a much more effective catalyst, available to the illicit phencyclidine chemist. Cars were raided for their platinum wire, as were college chemistry laboratories.

Increasingly, abusers synthesized their own supply in toilet tanks. These were ideal because they provided a ready supply of water and the porcelain could dissipate the heat. After the manufacture of phencyclidine became illegal, the choice of the toilet tank became fortuitous since incriminating evidence could be expeditiously flushed away while the police were still knocking on the door.

Because of its association with violent crimes and self destructive acts such as enucleation, immolation and suicide, PCP fell under the scrutiny of the Bureau of Narcotics and Dangerous Drugs. In 1967, its manufacture, sale and use became illegal under the provisions of the Comprehensive Drug Abuse, Prevention and Control Act. Because of the easy availability of its precursor and the ease with which the drug could be manufactured, the use of PCP continued unabated. As a result, in 1968, Congress passed the Psychotropic Substance Act. Among its provisions was a restriction on the sale of piperidine precursors. Because of the restriction of phencyclidine precursors, part-time chemists quickly reduced their activities and phencyclidine was less available to college students.

POPULATION AT RISK

Phencyclidine is generally a blue collar drug. Its typical abusers are white, blue-collar males living in industrial metropolitan areas in the Midwest and on the East and West Coasts. PCP use is greatest in New York City, Cleveland, Detroit, Chicago, Birmingham, St. Louis and Los Angeles. Abusers tend to have a high school or partial high school education. They are usually employed and work in unskilled or semiskilled jobs. This group of abusers knowingly buys PCP or its analogues for specific actions. PCP when knowingly purchased is vended as a powder to be dusted on marijuana cigarettes, or to be insufflated with crack cocaine, or to be ingested in nonmixed form.

A second set of abusers unknowingly buys PCP as an adulterant for another more expensive drug. The demographic profile of this type of unwitting abuser matches that of the target drug.

Phencyclidine is responsible for a small but discrete number of multiple and brutal assaultive crimes including rape and murder. Because of induced amnesia, many criminals have no recall of their acts. Many prosecutors' offices routinely test for PCP when particularly brutal crimes have been committed.

PHARMACOLOGY

Phencyclidine is a prototypical member of the group of drugs called the "dissociatives." All members of this group are arylcyclohexylamines. Their common chemical structure consists of the phenyl group, a piperidine group and a cyclohexyl ring (see Figure 10-1).

As shown in Figure 10-1, electron-dense regions in the aromatic ring and cyclohexyl ring are the source of specific cycloactive effects. Phencyclidine, along with the other dissociatives, has a cyclohexyl spine. This enables it to exist in rough equilibrium as two separate conformations having a phenyl grouping on either the axial or equatorial planes. Phencyclidine is in the active form when the phenyl group is in the plane of the axis. Dissociative activity is increased with the placement of an unsaturated bond in the triple ring structure. Potency can also be increased by replacing phenyl rings with thienyl groups or by adding a propyl sidechain. Nonpropyl sidechains, however, tend to weaken a dissociative, as does reduction in the number of rings and of saturating bonds.[9]

The most commonly used analogue is ketamine hydrochloride. It is a 2-O-chloralphenyl-1-2-methylaminecyclohexanome bicyclic. Its potency is markedly less than phencyclidine. The presence of side chains, in this case a chloride group, decreases its potency.

Another weak analogue, more similar in form to ketamine than phencyclidine, is PCE [N-ethyl-1-phenylcyclohexamine]. It is generally a byproduct of PCP production. It also occurs naturally as a weakly active metabolite of phencyclidine.

A fourth dissociative is PHP (1-[1-phenylcyclohexyl] pyrrolidine), another byproduct of phencyclidine production.

The phenyl group of PHP can be replaced with the thienyl group producing TCP (1-[2-thienlycyclohexyl] piperidine), the most potent of all dissociatives. It is approximately three- to five-times as potent as PCP.

Figure 10-2: Metabolites of Phencyclidine

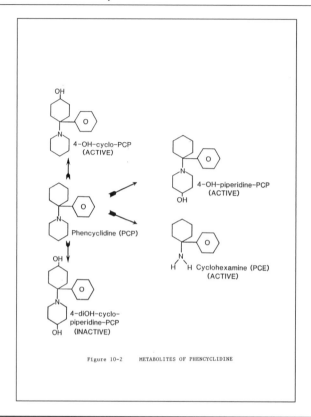

Figure 10-2   METABOLITES OF PHENCYCLIDINE

Among the weakest of analogues is PC [1-phenylcyclohexene]. It is most commonly formed in the combustion of PCP-dusted cigarettes.[10,11] Active and inactive metabolites are pictured in Figure 10-2.

The central effect of phencyclidine has been studied utilizing irradiated glucose. It has been found that the limbic cortex, the cingulate gyrus, the motor strip, the thalamus, the hippocampus, the antroventral thalamic projections, and the nucleus accumbens are areas of increased activity. The auditory system is a major area of decreased activity.

At the gross level, phencyclidine actions seem almost simplistic. At the microanatomical level, however, its actions become exceeding complex because of activity at multiple neurotransmitter receptor sites. Phencyclidine acts at acetylcholine, dopamine, opioid gamma-aminobutyric (GABA) and serotonin receptors. It also acts at the sigma receptor and two specific PCP receptor sites.[12]

Phencyclidine exhibits inhibitory actions at both central and peripheral cholinergic receptors. Because phencyclidine has the typical structure of an anticholinergic drug — a cationic head, phenyl group and large hydroxy group — it produces both nicotinic and muscarinic activities. Peripherally, it blocks potassium conduction and delays neurotransmitter release, depressing the amplitude of the striate muscle. This causes a decrease and rise in action potential and prolongs its duration. Other activity at the potassium channels also decreases the amount of acetylcholine-induced catecholamine release in the adrenal glands.

Although phencyclidine is indirectly competitive with nicotinic sites due to configurational changes of receptor sites, it is directly competitive with acetylcholine in muscarinic sites where it blocks cholinergic ionophores.[13] In addition, it blocks both pseudocholinesterase and butylcholinesterase activity. There seems to be no histamine cross-reactivity.[14]

Since chronic phencyclidine use was first noted to be associated with decreased levels of prolactin, a dopaminergic role was hypothesized. Later research demonstrated that there was a diminished response of thyroid stimulating hormone when stimulated by thyroid releasing hormone in the presence of phencyclidine. Phencyclidine has also been shown to mimic amphetamine-induced stereotypy and when combined with amphetamine, to enhance stereotypic effects.[15]

Both of the dopamine DA-2 blockers, haloperidol and pimozide, have been shown to reverse phencyclidine stereotypy and phencyclidine-induced prolactin suppression in rats. In treating phencyclidine psychosis, DA-2 specific neuroleptics such as pimozide and haloperidol have been shown superior to mixed DA-1/DA-2 neuroleptics such as chlorpromazine and fluphenazine.

Whereas amphetamines and cocaine stimulate the release of newly synthesized dopamine into the synaptic cleft, phencyclidine stimulates release of dopamine from the storage vesicles. Like the sympathomimetics, it also blocks dopaminergic reuptake, thus prolonging dopamine action and reducing recycling of the dopamine metabolite, homovanillic acid. In a manner similar to that of the sympathomimetics, the overall supply of dopamine is reduced. Further reducing the dopamine supply, phencyclidine inhibits dopamine accumulation in both the presynaptic vesicles and in the synaptasomes.

The addictive potential of phencyclidine is probably a function of its dopaminergic effects in the teleomesencephalic system including the pars compacta and the nucleus accumbens. Its dopamine activity stimulates the primary reward system and substitutes itself as a primary pseudodrive.[16]

Dopaminergic effects of phencyclidine on the primary drive centers of the brain seem to be mediated by opioids since naloxone blocks both euphoric and dysphoric effects. In addition, the anesthetic effects of phencyclidine and ketamine are due to their opiate-like properties. Phencyclidine and ketamine have both been shown to effect both μ and σ opioid receptors.[17] The μ-agonist, morphine, increases met-enkephalin-induced phencyclidine ataxia. This ataxia can be blocked over by naloxone. In addition, patients have been reported to exhibit a cross tolerance between meperidine, morphine or heroin and phencyclidine.[18]

Acutely, phencyclidine increases met-enkephalin. Methadone can suppress phencyclidine-induced behavior in rats and meperidine produces a similar response in humans. Ketamine produces an anesthetic effect that is as long-lived as that of morphine; phencyclidine produces an effect that is at least one-and-a-half times as long. Phencyclidine seems to work on the opioid system in a stimulatory depletion mode, much in the same way that it works on the dopaminergic system.

Phencyclidine also works upon GABA-minergic activity. The effects of acute phencyclidine intoxication have been recorded to be reduced with the benzodiazepines diazepam and chlordiazepoxide. However, more direct-acting GABA-minergic agonists such as barbiturates and methaqualone have not been effective in treating acute phencyclidine intoxication. It may be that the effect of the benzodiazepine B-Z receptor agonist might be a mere pseudo-effect, since PCP acts on a number of other receptors.

Phencyclidine may also act upon serotonin receptors since there is a cross-tolerance between phencyclidine, mescaline, psilocybin and lysergic acid.[19] Tests of rats' performance in two-level drug discrimination tests have demonstrated that these animals cannot distinguish phencyclidine from either LSD or mescaline. However, in contradistinction to the above evidence, post-LSD depression has been reported to respond only to fluoxetine, a relatively pure serotonergic antidepressant, whereas phencyclidine-withdrawal dysphoria has been reported to respond best to desipramine, a predominantly noradrenergic antidepressant. There have, however, been reports of geometricization, vivid visual hallucinations, depersonalization, derealization, astral projections, and synesthesia in phencyclidine patients. These hallmarks of LSD intoxication are not readily distinguished from PCP. REM-phase sleep studies have also been shown to produce similar tracings in both phencyclidine-intoxicated and LSD-intoxicated volunteers.

Three unique receptors have been found to be utilized by phencyclidine. The first is a σ-receptor, a possible opioid receptor which is insensitive to naloxone.[20] It does, however, bind with the experimental opioid drug SKF-10,047. Haloperidol antagonizes this receptor whereas chlorpromazine and other phenothiazines are generally ineffective here. Functions of this receptor site and its hypothesized ligand are unknown.

The two other phencyclidine receptors are PCP-specific. One is a high-affinity binding site located within the NDMA (N-methyl-D-aspartate) receptor channel. It is stimulated by glutamate but irreversibly antagonized by metaphit. This site is noninteractive with haloperidol, chlorpromazine, pimozide, naloxone or SKF-10,047. This receptor is located throughout the brain, including the hippocampus and its projections, as well as the cingulate gyrus, corpus callosum, inferior colliculi, locus coeruleus, medulla oblongata and anterior pons.

The second PCP-specific receptor site is one of lower infinity. It is reportedly noninteractive with metaphit, naloxone, haloperidol and chlorpromazine. Thus far, no antagonist has been found but it is known to be agonized by N-allylnormetazocine. The distribution of this low-affinity PCP receptor site has not yet been determined.[21-23]

DIAGNOSIS

Presentation of phencyclidine intoxication varies according to the dosage. Low dosage usually tends to produce symptoms of anticholinergic intoxication. Patients with these symptoms are best remembered by Sir William Osler's triad: they are mad as a hatter, red as a beet, and dry as a bone. At moderate doses, the opiate receptors seem to be most interactive and the patient tends to be in a dream-like state with various degrees of anesthesia. At higher dosages, dopaminergic systems seem to predominate and the patient may be paranoid, confused or hallucinating. There are, however, eight symptoms which tend to be present at all levels of intoxication. They are best remembered by the mnemonic RED DANES (see Figure 10-3).[24]

Figure 10-3: Mnemonic Symptoms of Acute Phencyclidine Intoxication

R   (Rage)

E   (Erythema)

D   (Dilated pupils)

D   (Delusions)

A   (Amnesia)

N   (Nystagmus in the horizontal plane)

E   (Excitation)

S   (Skin dry)

Other reported symptoms include ataxia, dysarthria, hyperacusis, prolonged hypertensive episodes, tonic-clonic seizures and rigidity. Prolonged seizures under PCP do not seem to produce deleterious effect. This might be due to phencyclidine action at the high-affinity PCP receptor, which acts to prevent neuronal cellular death by exhibiting lysosome-induced cell death during periods of anoxia.

TREATMENT

Since phencyclidine works at a number of sites, there is unfortunately no specific antidote for acute intoxication as in most other drugs of abuse.[25,26] Some authors have urged that a variable antidotal model be used based on the hypothesis that specific symptom clusters are caused by a predominance of activity at one specific neurotransmitter system.[27] However, using the biopsychiatric model, specific symptom clusters can be treated by appropriate pharmacological intervention based on positive symptom presentation rather than trying to ascertain dosage levels.

Since PCP has anticholinergic activities, it can produce horizontal nystagmus, red dry skin, photodermititis and mydriasis. EKG if available can often show T-wave flattening, T-wave inversion, ST depression and widening of the QRS interval with occasional U waves, circus rhythms and Q waves. There might also be rare atonic bladder and ileus. In this case, treatment is the same for anticholinergic overdose: physostigmine salicylate 2 mg. intramuscularly every 20 to 30 minutes until QRS interval contracts to less than 10 mm., or until the atonic bladder or abdominal ileus is relieved.[28,29]

Other anticholinergic actions include hypertensive crisis secondary to phencyclidine actions upon the adrenal medulla. By blocking cholinergic receptors, large amounts of norepinephrine are released from the medulla. To counteract these effects, 1 mg. of the beta-blocker propanol is introduced intravenously by titration. If the patient is asthmatic, propanol is contraindicated. In this latter case, dioxide 2.5 mg. per kg. can be given intravenously in a 20 to 30 second infusion.[30]

Dopaminergic effects include psychosis, paranoid agitation, delusions, and occasional mutism. Other symptoms include seizures, myoclonus, stereotypy, hypersalivation and hyperreflexia. This symptom complex is produced by stimulation of the DA-2 receptor. In this case, DA-2 antagonists such as haloperidol, 5 mg. every 20 minutes intramuscularly should be prescribed.[31,32] Generally, haloperidol will block all of the above symptoms between the third and fifth dose. A recent case report has indicated similar efficacy with risperidone.

At very high, nearly lethal dosage ranges, opioid activity is occasionally seen. The patient is totally anesthetized to pain and can manifest fever in excess of 103°F. There is encopresis and enuresis. Hyporeflexia and hypotension with cardiac arrhythmias are seen. Opisthotonos manifests itself and convulsions may continue to occur. At this point, the prognosis is poor. Researchers have reported success using naloxone but it cannot be recommended since naloxone can cause hyperthermia in low-dose phencyclidine intoxication, and hypothermia in high-dose phencyclidine intoxication. More haloperidol can be given in spite of the opioid presentation because of dopaminergic interaction with the opioid system. Hypothermia can also be reduced with alcohol sponges and cooling blankets.[33,34]

A major component of acute intervention involves "ion trapping." Ion trapping is a concept which utilizes the relative insolubility of ionized phencyclidine to remove it from the systemic circulation. To accomplish this, contents of the gastrointestinal tract are acidified and the phencyclidine is isolated and sequestered. Ingested phencyclidine can be sequestered in the gastrointestinal tract by instilling magnesium sulfate into the stomach via nasogastric tube at a dosage of 0.3 g. per kg. In this manner, the relatively inactive ionized state will be maintained and fecal elimination will be facilitated.

When phencyclidine is used in any form, ascorbic acid 1000 mg. intramuscularly every 6 hours can be used to trap the ionized form of phencyclidine into the bladder. Ascorbic acid acidifies the urine and renders ionized phencyclidine incapable of reentering the circulatory system. To increase the elimination of ionized phencyclidine from the urinary tract, furosemide 40 mg. intramuscularly combined with a 0.9 N sodium chloride drip at a maximally tolerated delivery rate will also remove phencyclidine from the system. Ascorbic acid apparently has mild antipsychotic properties of its own in phencyclidine intoxication and acts synergistically with haloperidol.[35] Without ascorbic acid, the urinary route accounts for only 9 percent of total elimination of phencyclidine with a renal clearance of 0.3 liters per min. Utilizing ascorbic acid at the above dosage can increase clearance to 3.0 ml. per min. with a urinary clearance of almost 70 percent.

Long-term phencyclidine addiction predisposes a patient to a post-withdrawal dysphoria. In this state the patient is depressed, anhedonic and anergic. There is insomnia and relative anorexia. Initial studies report success with desipramine 200 to 300 mg. every day. If the patient presents initially intoxicated, desipramine should not be initiated upon presentation because of interactive anticholinergic effects between this tricyclic antidepressant and phencyclidine. Desipramine may be safely started, however, after two to three days of drug-free state.[36]

In treating the pregnant or nursing mother, phencyclidine causes several problems. Children whose mothers have abused phencyclidine on an infrequent basis have been reported to have hypertonicity, increased startle reflex, spasticity, and tremor. In many cases, the baby presents with icteric sclera or frank jaundice. There have been several case reports of children with mongoloid features, although they did not possess trisomy 18.[37,38] After detoxification has been accomplished and post withdrawal depression treated, there remains the problem of investigating the reason for the mother's abuse. Patients who have knowingly and chronically abused phencyclidine tend to be rebellious yet hard-working women. A common complain is that "the system is against me." They generally tend to be passive individuals with suppressed rage who occasionally explode. There is also a high degree of character disorder, which is higher than most other drug abusing populations. Therapy should focus on empowerment and teaching the patient how to emerge from a self-perceived helpless state. Control of aggression is also a hallmark of intervention with this sort of patient.

Because of their passivity punctuated by extreme aggressivity, phencyclidine patients do not do well in nonstructured groups such as Narcotics Anonymous. They perform well, however, in psychotherapeutic interventions run by a psychiatrist experienced with this type of patient. Since phencyclidine is not known to be addicting, the patient can be returned safely to his former environment without the same risks seen in alcohol, cocaine or heroin abusing populations.

TYPICAL CASE PRESENTATION

The patient was a 24-year-old, white female who was brought to the emergency room by a friend. She was extremely disoriented and agitated. The friend said that the patient had been smoking crack cocaine and "then she just freaked out." Vital signs revealed an axillary temperature of 101°F, a heart rate of 92 beats per min., and a blood pressure of 150/110 mm. Hg. Because of the clear history of cocaine intoxication, she was triaged to the hospital's chemical dependency service (CDS).

The internist covering the CDS took the patient's history from her friend since the patient was belligerent when he spoke to her. The patient reportedly had been smoking crack cocaine at the rate of 5 to 6 "rocks" per day, five days per week for three years. There was no history of a similar explosive episode. The friend did note, however, a progressive history of anorexia, anergia and social withdrawal.

Superficial examination revealed a highly agitated, muscular, young, white female. She was flushed but did not appear diaphoretic. Pupils were dilated. She appeared to be responding to unseen visual stimuli. Movements were jerky and somewhat repetitive. The initial diagnoses were then made. These included: cocaine-precipitated brief reactive psychosis, acute phencyclidine intoxication, and cocaine psychosis. The internist attempted a brief exam but he was struck in the chest by the patient.

A psychiatrist was called. The patient was subdued by two teams of aides. When she was immobilized, she was injected with haloperidol 5 mg. intramuscularly in an exposed thigh. Within 15 minutes the patient demonstrated a noticeable response. She was still agitated but neither belligerent nor assaultive. She allowed herself to be injected with a second dose of haloperidol and was more pliable. At that time, a physical examination revealed horizontal nystagmus, hyperreflexia, myoclonus and absent bowel sounds. Skin was flushed and dry. Pupils were extremely

Table 10-1: Phencyclidine: Relationship between Specific Symptoms and Dosage

DOSAGE	SYMPTOMS	
1 to 5 mg.	Agitation Amnesia Anxiety Ataxia Conceptual disorganization	Excitation Hallucinations, visual Hyperacusis Photophobia
6 to 10 mg.	Amnesia Anxiety Conceptual disorganization Confusion Delusions Fever Hallucinations, visual Hypertension Hypersalivation	Hyperreflexia Mutism Myoclonus Stereotypy Stupor Tachycardia Violence
11+ mg.	Amnesia Arrythmia Coma Convulsions Delusions Diaphoresis Encopresis Excitement Fever	Hallucinations, auditory Hallucinations, visual Hyporeflexia Hypotension Mutism Opisthotonus Violence

dilated. Heart rate was 95 beats per min. with occasional skipped beats. A urine sample was then obtained for toxicology analysis, though a working diagnosis was made of acute phencyclidine intoxication of approximately 10 mg. (see Table 10-1).

The initial step was elimination of the phencyclidine with "ion trapping." She was injected with 1000 mg. ascorbic acid intramuscularly, followed by furosemide 40 mg. intramuscularly. An IV line of 0.9 N saline was begun and run at 120 cc per hr. During this procedure, the patient began to decompensate and a third intramuscular injection of haloperidol was administered, 45 minutes after initial dose.

An abdominal flat plate was obtained from a portable X-ray unit. It confirmed the presence of ileus. This was treated with physostigmine salicylate 2 mg. intramuscularly. This dose was repeated in thirty minutes with good result. During this time, the heart rate increased to 100 beats per min. with periods of arrhythmia. Blood pressure was now 160/120 mm. Hg. This was treated with propanol 1 mg. intravenously in a 20-second infusion.

The patient responded to the protocol and was transferred to the inpatient detoxification unit. There her IV line was continued for 24 hours. She received ascorbic acid 1000 mg. every 8 hours during this time. Haloperidol was prescribed 5 mg. by mouth every 6 hours for 24 hours, and then gradually decreased over a two-day period. During this time, the patient began demonstrating depression and cocaine craving. It was determined by the staff that her addiction was to cocaine and that phencyclidine toxicity was due to involuntary ingestion. She was therefore transferred to an inpatient drug rehabilitation unit for treatment of cocaine addiction and withdrawal.

NOTES

1. Giannini AJ. PCP: detecting the abuser. Med Aspects Human Sexuality. 1987; **21(1)**:100.

2. Giannini AJ, Loiselle RH, Giannini MC et al. The dissociative. Med Psychiatry 1987; **3(3)**:197.

3. Giannini AJ, Castellani S. A case of phenylcyclohexyl pyrrolidine (PHP) intoxication treated with physostigmine. Clin Toxicol 1982; **19**:505-508.

4. Allen AC, Robles J, Dovenski W, Calderon S. PCP: a review of synthetic methods for forensic clandestine investigation. Forensic Sci Int 1993; **61(2-3)**:85-100.

5. Gibb RP, Cockerham H, Goldfogel GA, Lawson GM, Raisys VA. substance abuse testing of urine by GC/MS in scanning mode evaluated by proficiency studies, TLC/GC, and EMIT. J Forensic Sci 1993; **38(1)**:124-33.

6. Sneath TC, Jain NC. Evaluation of phencyclidine by EMIT d.a.u. utilizing ETS analyzer and a 25-ng/mL cutoff. J Anal Toxicol 1992; **16(2)**:48-51.

7. Schwarzhoff R, Cody JT. The effects of adulterating agents on FPIA analysis of urine for drugs of abuse. J Anal Toxicol 1980; **17(1)**:14-7.

8. Davis BM, Beach HR. The effect of 1-arylcyclohexylamine (Sernyl) on twelve normal volunteers. J Ment Sci 1960; **106**:912-924.

9. Synder SH. Phencyclidine. Nature. 1980; **285**:355-356.

10. Giannini AJ, Loiselle RH, Malone DM, et al. Treatment of PHP (phenylhexylcyclopyrrolidine) psychosis with haloperidol. Clin Toxicol 1985; **23**:185-189.

11. Cook CE. Pyrolytic characteristics, pharmacokinetics, and bioavailability of smoked heroin, cocaine, phencyclidine and methamphetamine. NIDA Res Monogr 1991; **115**:6-23.

12. Weissman AD, Casanova MF, Kleinman JE, De Souza EB. PCP and sigma receptors in brain are not altered after repeated exposure to PCP in humans. Neuropsychopharmacology 1991; **4(2)**:95-102.

13. Albuquerque TX, Aguayo LG, Warnick JE, et al. Interactions of phencyclidine with ion channels of nerve and muscle behavioral implications. Fed Proc 1983; **42**:2852-2859.

14. Giannini AJ, Price WA, Giannini MC, Lazurus HD, Loiselle RH. Absence of response to H-1 blockade in phencyclidine toxicity. J Clin Pharmacol 1986; **26**:716-717.

15. Castellani S, Giannini AJ, Adams PM. Effects of naloxone, metenkephalin and morphine on phencyclidine induced behavior in the rat. Psychopharmacology 1982; **78**:76-80.

16. Giannini AJ, Drug abuse and depression. Catecholamine depletion suggested as biological tie between cocaine withdrawal and depression. Natl Inst Drug Abuse Notes 1987; **2(2)**:5.

17. Wolfe SA Jr, De Souza ED. Sigma and phencyclidine receptors in the brain-endocrine-immune axis. NIDA Res Monogr 1993; **133**:95-123.

18. Giannini AJ, Loiselle RH, Price WA, et al. Comparison of chlorpromazine and meperidine in the treatment of phencyclidine psychosis. J Clin Psychiatry 1985; **46(4)**:52-55.

19. Giannini AJ, Loiselle RH, Graham BH, Folts DJ. Behavioral response to buspirone in cocaine and phencyclidine withdrawal. J Subst Abuse Treat 1993; **10(6)**:523-7.

20. Contreras PC, Gray NM, DiMaggio DA, Bremer ME, Bussom JA. Isolated and characterization of an endogenous ligand for the PCP and sigma receptors from porcine, rat, and human tissue. NIDA Res Monogr 1993; **133**:207-22

21. Comptom RP, Contreras PC, O'Donohue TL, et al. The N-methyl-d-aspartate antagonist, 2-amino-7-phosphonoheptanoate, produces phencyclidine-like behavioral effects in rats. Eur J Pharmacol. (In press.)

22. Tamminga CA, Tuniomoto K, Chase TN et al: PCP-induced alterations in cerebral glucose utilization. Synapse 1987; **1**:497,504.
23. Zukin SR, Javitt DC. Phencyclidine receptor binding as a probe of NMDA receptor functioning: implications for drug abuse research. NIDA Res Monogr 1993; **133**:1-2.
24. Giannini AJ. Red Danes. Primary Care/Emergency Decisions 1987; **3(4)**:53.
25. Moriarty RW. Managing phencyclidine toxicity. Drug Ther 1978; **14(6)**:166-172.
26. Aronow R, Done AK. Phencyclidine overdose. An emerging concept of management. J AM Coll Emergency Physicians 1978; **7**:56-59.
27. Giannini AJ, Giannini MC, Price WA. Antidotal strategies in phencyclidine intoxication. Int J Psych Med 1984; **4(4)**:513.
28. Castellani S. Adams PM, Giannini AJ. Physostigmine treatment of acute phencyclidine intoxication. J Clin Psychiatry 1982; **43(5)**:10-11.
29. Castellani S, Giannini AJ, Adams PM. Physostigmine and haloperidol treatment of acute phencyclidine intoxication. Am J Psychiatry. 1982; **139**:508.
30. Castellani S, Giannini AJ, Boeringa P, et al. PCP intoxication-assessment of possible antidotes. Clin Toxicol 1982; **19(5)**:505.
31. Giannini AJ, Eighan MD, Giannini MC, et al. Comparison of haloperidol and chlorpromazine in the treatment of phencyclidine psychosis: Role of the DA-2 receptor. J Clin Pharmacol 1980; **61**:401-405.
32. Giannini AJ, Nageotte C, Loiselle RH et al. Comparison of chlorpromazine, haloperidol and pimozide in the treatment of phencyclidine psychosis: Role of the DA-2 receptor. Clin Toxicol 1985; **22**:573.
33. Giannini AJ, Price WA. Management of acute intoxication. Med Times 1985; **113(9)**:43.
34. Milhorn HT, Jr. Diagnosis and management of phencyclidine intoxication. Am Fam Physician 1991; **43(4)**:1293-302.
35. Giannini AJ. Augmentation of haloperidol by ascorbic acid in phencyclidine intoxication. Am J Psychiatry 1987; **144**:1207-1209.
36. Giannini AJ, Malone DA, Giannini MC, et al. Treatment of chronic cocaine and phencyclidine abuse with desipramine. J Clin Pharmacol 1986; **26**:211.

37. Van Dyke DC, Fox AA. Fetal drug exposure and its possible implications for learning in the preschool and school-age population. J Learn Disabil 1990; **23(3)**:160-3.

38. Rahbar F, Fomufod A, Whiate D. Westney LS. Impact of intrauterine exposure to phencyclidine (PCP) and cocaine on neonates. J Natl Med Assoc 1993; **85(5)**:349-52.

CHAPTER 11

PSYCHEDELICS

The psychedelics, also called hallucinogenic agents, are drugs capable of unique and complex effects. They create multiple distortions and hallucinogenic experiences which can encompass all the senses. Sensory distortions may occur independently or simultaneously, or may cross so that the user can hear colors or smell sounds. This latter effect, called "synesthesia," is a characteristic feature of LSD but may occur with any psychedelic agent. The attraction of psychedelics includes their short-lived actions, near-immediate onset and lack of addictive potential.

While psychedelic agents can precipitate underlying psychosis, their effects are generally not permanent. The psychedelic-driven hallucinations are generally readily distinguishable from schizophrenic and organic hallucinatory states. Generally, the abuser can distinguish between the distorted internal "reality" and the external reality experience. Unlike the schizophrenic (and like Alice in her *Adventures through the Looking Glass*), psychedelic abusers can easily skip across the twin experiential planes or they can co-exist in the planes simultaneously.[1]

It has been previously noted by the author that the psychedelic abuser is in the same situation as the audience at the cinema. Members of the audience may observe the film on the screen as well as the decor within the theater. In like fashion, the psychedelic abusers can experience reality in a similar way, except the screen exists solely within the theater of the mind. On the screen are viewed idiosyncratic images. These images, though internally derived, are influenced by the external environment in the same manner as is the sleeper whose dreams are shaped by a television that has been left on in the same room.[2]

LABORATORY TESTING

The most frequently utilized and detected psychedelic is lysergic acid diethylamide (LSD). LSD and its metabolites can be detected for longer periods in urine samples than in serum samples. If the urine or serum sample is not analyzed immediately, it must be stored in a cool, dark place since LSD decomposes in the presence of moderate light and elevated room temperatures. Detection is always difficult because microscopically low doses of LSD are used to achieve mind-altering experiences. Therefore, compounds are present in the pica-gram range. Preferred testing procedures are by radioimmunoassay (RIA) which also detects cross-reactive metabolites. Gas chromatography/mass spectrometry (GC/MS) can also be used for detection in quantitative analysis.[3]

Methylenedioxymethamphetamine (MDMA), also known as ecstasy or "X," is similar to amphetamine and methamphetamine. Qualitative screens can be conducted by immunoassay with Abbot A/M or Abuscreen/HSM. Occasionally it can be done by gas chromatography. It should be noted, however, that in using immunoassay, LSD cross-reacts with MDMA and with other amphetamine compounds.[4]

HISTORY

Psychedelic tradition has two roots: the first comes from the pre-Columbian Americas and the second from the Eurasian land mass. The first psychedelic for which there is some evidence of use was fly agaric, a toxic mushroom known scientifically as *Amanita muscaria*. Anthropological evidence indicates that this was used 3,000 to 4,000 years ago contemporaneously in central Asia, northern India, Siberia and pharaonic Egypt.

A second and later source of psychedelic compound was rye rust, which produces the ergot alkaloids. In preclassical Greece in Elusia near Athens, the Elusian rites were practiced. The rite celebrates the return of Ceres' daughter, Persephone, to the world of nature from the underworld home of her husband, Pluto. Visitors to this festival drank a mixture of wine, flour, herbs and ergot. Ergot was later compounded for use at the hospitals of classical Greece. The psychedelic compounds, which were named "aesklepions" after Aesclepius, produced hallucinations in the patients. The Greek physicians would administer askelpions and then make diagnoses based on the patient's self-described hallucinations.

Rye rust also produced many instances of "demonic possession" in northern European villages throughout the Middle Ages. Outbreaks of rye rust and the resultant ingestion of the grain would produce a disease that was called St. Anthony's Fire. It was accompanied by painful burning sensations and visual hallucinations.

It is hypothesized that nutmeg was used to produce hallucinatory experiences in the late Renaissance and Baroque periods. Nutmeg was used as a symbolic device in many paintings and may have produced the bizarre works of Hieronymous Bosch, as well as added an other-worldly quality to some of the paintings of Paolo Ucello.

Psychedelic use was more widespread in the pre-Columbian Americas. The Toltecs and their Aztec successors utilized psilocybin mushrooms at the coronation of the kings. The Aztecs also used morning glory seeds containing LSD precursors. These were utilized by the priest to obtain the compliance of his sacrificial victim. In North America, peyote buttons continued to be used by the Native Americans in the Sierra Madres, the Great Plains and the Sonora Desert. In South America, the flower *Anadenanthera* provided seeds which were ground and insufflated. These seeds were used ritualistically for war, hunting and marriage. They were later adopted by Spanish crewmen during Columbus's later voyages.

In the nineteenth century, Henry Havelock-Ellis experimented with mescaline and published his results, the first semicontrolled study of the psychedelic agents, in his "contemporary science" series of books.

In nineteenth century America, safrole, a mild psychedelic found in sassafras oil, was used in sassafras tea, root beer and sarsaparilla. Its use continued in reduced form until the 1960's when it was declared an illegal substance due to its carcinogenic, but not psychedelic, properties.

In the twentieth century, the influence of psychedelics upon visual art was seen with George Bracque and Pablo Picasso who may have written *The Cubist Manifesto* while influenced by mescaline. A flattening effect known as geometricization is reflected in cubist art and is a noted effect of mescaline.

Modern psychedelic culture is thought to have been generated in 1938 in Basel, Switzerland. It was there that Albert Hoffman at Sandoz Laboratories synthesized D-lysergic acid diethylamide-25. In 1943, Hoffman accidently absorbed LSD through his skin and later experienced visual distortions while riding his bicycle. Four years after this, Werner Stoll published a series of LSD case reports.

Psychedelics became more popular in the 1950's when Aldous Huxley and Humphrey Osmond engaged in a series of unsupervised experiments with mescaline. Huxley published and popularized its effect in *Doors of Perception*. He later described his subjective sensations at the 1958 annual convention of the American Psychiatric Association.

In the 1960's, a Harvard University experimental project under the guidance of Timothy Leary and Richard Albert lead to the public attention of their experiences in *The Psychedelic Experience: A Manual Based on the Tibetan Book of the Dead*. A similar popularization effort was published by Ken Kesey, who after participating in a similar research program at Stanford University, incorporated his psychedelic experiences in *One Flew Over the Cuckoo's Nest*. Kesey's later experiences were further popularized by Tom Wolfe in his novel, *The Electric Kool-Aid Acid Test*. Also in the 1960's and 1970's, Carlos Castaneda published a series of popular semi-fictional novels. In these novels, he was led on mystic revelations and fantastic explorations with an Native American guide, Don Juan, under the influence of a psychedelic substance. These publications tended to create a subculture based on the use of psychedelic drugs, Eastern mysticism, hedonistic philosophy and sexual liberation.

The movement continued until the 1970's when it imploded because its leaders could not sustain a viable culture. Timothy Leary was reported to be locked up in a basement in a psychotic state by the Black Panther, Eldridge Cleaver, in Algeria. The Altamont rock festival of 1970 included the death of a patron at the hands of a cue-stick-wielding Hell's Angel during a Rolling Stones performance. Contemporaneous to this time, the Haight-Ashbury district became the site of numerous murders under the influence of amphetamine addicts ("speed kills"), driving out the gentler, more introspective psychedelic trippers. Finally, there was the coup de grace which came about during the ritualistic murders of Sharon Tate and her friends by the psychedelic-driven followers of Charles Manson (*Helter Skelter*). By the time the rock opera paean to psychedelia, *Hair*, was produced as a motion picture, no one came and no one cared.

POPULATION AT RISK

Psychedelic drug use peaked in the late 1960's and nearly disappeared by the late 1970's. Currently, its popularity has undergone a resurgence. The National Institute of Drug Abuse reports that while the percentage of high school seniors using psychedelics has increased from 4.9 to 5.3 percent, the percentage of eighth grade students has increased from 3.8 to 5.3 percent. Psychedelics are also increasing in popularity among college students, college-educated workers and blue-collar workers.[5]

Teenagers apparently use LSD because it is relatively inexpensive and perceived to be a safe drug. Teenagers and young adults are increasingly using psychedelic drugs and materials in association with "rave" parties. These parties are commercial events in which pre-recorded technomusic, hyperkinectic dancing, psychedelic drugs, and nonalcoholic beverages are provided.[6,7]

Among middle-age devotees of psychedelics, MDMA (ecstasy) is the drug of choice. MDMA is a drug which uniquely provides increased libidinal awareness in both sexes, sustained penile erection in the male, and a perception of physical merging with one's lover. It is a popular drug which, despite its expense, is often used by overworked, highly stressed and urbanized professionals.[8]

PHARMACOLOGY

The psychedelic drugs act at serotonergic, as well as dopaminergic, receptor sites. All psychedelics have either an indolethylamine or phenylethylamine nucleus.[9] Dimethyltryptophan and psilocybin are constructed about an indolethylamine nucleus, whereas mescaline has a phenylethylamine nucleus. LSD, interestingly, incorporates both indolethylamine and phenylethylamine nuclei into its structure. Indolethylamine psychedelics inhibit serotonergic neuron firing in the pontine raphe nuclei, whereas only indolamine psychedelics agonize 5-HT_1A autoreceptors.

All psychedelics, however, stimulate 5-HT_2 post synaptic receptors. These 5-HT_2 receptors are located throughout the cerebral cortex as well as the claustrum facial nucleus, nucleus accumbens, nucleus tractus solitarius, and the piriform cortex. The 5-HT receptors seem to be the etiological factor in the development of the cognitive and sensory distortion produced by the indolethylalamine psychedelics.[10] It is hypothesized that 5-HT_1A receptor activity distorts the balance between 5-HT_2 and 5-HT_1A receptors. The unique sensation of synesthesia (cross-sensory distortion) may be a function of LSD's combined action on both 5-HT_1A and 5-HT_2 receptors.[11]

The action of psychedelic agents is not limited to the central nervous system. This may account for peripheral serotonergic manifestations such as diarrhea, diaphoresis and mydriasis. LSD is metabolized into the liver to form 2-oxy-lysergic acid diethylamide. It is distributed throughout the kidneys, liver and lungs. The minimum effective dose of LSD (i.e., a dose that causes nonspecific perceptual distortions) is 5 μg, and the minimum hallucinogenic dose (i.e., dose that causes hallucinations) is 20 to 40 μg. Although there is no reported toxic range in humans, it approaches 5 μg. per kg. in rhesus monkeys. The half-life of LSD is approximately three hours.

Mescaline is an alkaloid: 3,4,5-trimethoxyphenylethylamine. In addition to its serotonergic activity, it stimulates adenylate cyclase activity of dopaminergic receptors in the anterior limbic and auditory cortices. Absorption is rapid, although hallucinations may not occur for up to five hours after ingestion. It is 30 percent metabolized in the liver by N-acetylation and deamination of side chains. It is 90 percent protein bound and excreted renally. Concentration is in the liver, spleen and kidneys.

Methylenedioxymethamphetamine (MDMA or ecstasy) is a synthetic derivative of amphetamine that is produced by adding a dioxymethylene ring to the benzene portion of the amphetamine molecule. This derivative combines action of both the psychedelics and the sympathomimetics. It acts at α-receptors, stimulating both adrenergic and noradrenergic neurons at both central and peripheral receptor sites. In addition, it increases serotonergic release and blocks reuptake. Effective dosage is between 100 and 150 mg. orally. Onset occurs within 20 to 40 minutes after ingestion with a plateau state lasting between 3 to 4 hours. After-effects can last 24 hours. Some evidence indicates that chronic MDMA use may irreversibly damage central serotonergic axons.

Psilocybin is an indolethylamine and acts upon 5-HT$_1$A. Unlike mescaline, it does not mediate activity at 5-HT$_1$A autoreceptors. There is some evidence that psilocybin also has particular affinity for the color receptors in the retina. Psilocybin is thought to produce psychoactive effects at the serotonergic pontine raphe nuclei. It is rapidly absorbed and metabolized in the liver by oxidation. Onset of action is within 15 to 30 minutes. Activity continues for approximately 5 to 8 hours.[12]

Nutmeg is a complex mixture of a variety of psychoactive compounds including lysergol, geraniol, saffrol, eugenol, and borneol. These act at many sites in the central nervous system as well as at the adrenal medullae. In addition, nutmeg contains myristicene, which contributes atropinic effects and has an effect similar to that of ipecac. Hallucinations occur after ingestion of one whole nutmeg or 5 grams of grated nutmeg. The minimal lethal dose is 10 grams of grated nutmeg or 2 whole nutmegs. This is usually due to cardiac arrhythmias compounded by uncontrolled emesis.

N,N-dimethyltryptophan (DMT) acts physiologically in a fashion similar to LSD. Its onset is quite rapid with effects being experienced within seconds of injection or smoking. These plateau rapidly with a duration of approximately 30 minutes. Minimum dosage is 1 mg. per kg. with lethality approached at 10 to 15 mg. per kg. In addition to central effects, there are sympathomimetic effects. Metabolism is hepatic by a variety of mechanisms.

DIAGNOSIS

The psychedelics have both generalized diagnostic characteristics as well as "signature" symptoms for each element in this group. Acutely, there are sensory distortions and hallucinations. These hallucinations can be dynamic or static and seem to exists against a backlit background. In many cases, the patient describes visual hallucinations superimposed on a background imprinted with reticular netting, spiral tunneling or receding walls. There can be movement in visual fields so that the figures explode towards the viewer. At times, figures may seem to "breathe" or "pulse." These subjective effects may be accompanied by diaphoresis, dizziness, emesis, hypothermia, mydriasis, pilomotor erection and resting tremor.[2,13]

LSD uniquely produces synesthesia, otherwise known as cross-sensory distortions. It can produce unique hallucinations in which a particular perceived element shares many sensations (e.g., "smelling a loud wet cinnamon color"). Psilocybin creates intensification of color. As one hyperbolic psilocybin abuser described, "I saw 5,000 shades of red, 1,000 shades of green and 10,000 shades of blue." Mescaline is associated with flattening and geometricization of figures (e.g., cubist figures).

Nutmeg intoxication produces visual hallucinations associated with emesis, arrhythmias and abdominal pain. Chronic use of nutmeg will produce bilateral pain at the level of the kidneys. Dimethyltryptophan is associated with elevated blood pressure, hallucinations and sensory distortions sometimes accompanied by the sensation of merging with animate or inanimate objects. Ecstasy can produce jaw clenching, bruxism and intense euphoria. Unique visual distortions include a shining or shimmering patina on objects within the visual field. There is also extreme diaphoresis and ataxia associated with increased psychomotor activity.[13,14]

Chronic use of psychedelics can produce depression which may lead to suicide. Long after psychedelic drug use has occurred, there may be a spontaneous recurrence of any one or more elements of the specific drug-induced psychosis. Thus the previous intoxication can exert effects many years later. This phenomenon is know as a "flashback" and most commonly occurs after chronic hallucinogenic drug use. Most common flashbacks include prolongation of the after-image or white flashes in the peripheral vision. Other specific elements such as image flattening with mescaline use, or shimmering effects of objects with MDMA use, may recur. Flashbacks may be repetitive but they tend to disappear after one year of drug discontinuance.[15]

TREATMENT

Acute intoxication can be treated by supportive measures. These include reassurance and a low-stimulus environment. If anxiety occurs, it can be treated with diazepam 5 to 10 mg. intramuscularly or, if accompanied by tachycardia or other sympathomimetic effects, with propranolol 10 to 20 mg. orally or 0.5 to 1.0 mg. intravenously at a rate of 1 mg. per min. to a maximum of 6 mg.

Initial psychotic behavior can be treated with haloperidol 1 to 5 mg. intramuscularly. Persistent psychosis can be treated with risperdone 1 to 3 mg. every day, four times a day orally. Risperdone is a preferred antipsychotic because of its specific antagonism of $5-HT_2$ receptors.

Pharmacological treatment of psychedelic-induced depression includes prescription of a serotonin reuptake inhibitor. Preliminary studies indicate positive responses to paroxetine 20 mg. every day, three times a day, or fluoxetine 20 to 40 mg. every day, twice a day. Both of these antidepressants are presumed to exert their effects by blocking inhibiting neuronal serotonin reuptake.[16,17]

In addition to pharmacological treatment, outpatient chemical dependency treatment should be sought in a supportive environment based on a 12-step program. When advising the patient to develop a drug-free life style, the patient should be encouraged to talk through and emotionally discharge his perceptually unique experiences. These patients generally see themselves as creative individuals. Resistance to treatment occurs when the person equates giving up psychedelic abuse with giving up his creativity.

TYPICAL CASE PRESENTATION

A twenty-four-year-old white male was brought to the emergency room by his female companion who gave a brief history and left. She said that she had returned to her apartment after classes to find the patient staring fixedly at his right hand.

He was triaged to the psychiatry resident. Vital signs were unremarkable. The patient was distracted and apparently responding to unseen objects or persons. In walking to his cubicle, the patient appeared unsteady and was placed in a wheelchair. He responded to questions with brief nonsequitors and sentence fragments. He passively submitted to a physical examination which revealed only mydriasis and resting tremor. The working diagnosis of "psychosis rule-out catatonia" was made. However, a stat serum and urine drug screen was ordered.

While waiting for the drug screen, the patient became anxious and tried to climb over the rails of the cot. The resident returned to find an extremely anxious and diaphoretic patient. He ordered lorazepam 2 mg. intramuscularly on a stat basis which partially calmed the patient. This dose was repeated in 40 minutes when the agitation returned. Shortly after the second dose, the urine screen came back positive for LSD.

The patient was then transferred to the hospital's drug-rehabilitation unit. There he was placed in a seclusion room and observed every 30 minutes. He fell asleep after approximately four hours. In the morning, the patient was alert and oriented. After admitting the use of LSD to staff, he signed out against medical advise.

NOTES

1. Giannini AJ. Afterword. In: PJ Farmer, Red Orc's Rage. NY: Tor Publishing, 1991, pp. 279-282.
2. Giannini AJ. Inward the mind's I: Treatment of LSD flashbacks and hallucinations. Psychiatric Ann 1994; **24(3)**:134.
3. Kysilka R, Wurst M, Paćakov V, Sutlìk K, Hăskovec L. High-performance liquid chromatographic determination of hallucinogenic indolamines with simultaneous UV photometric and voltametric detection. J Chromatogr 1985; **320(2)**:414-20.
4. Musacchio JM, Klein M, Canoll PD. Dextromethorphan and sigma ligands: common sites but diverse effects. Life Sci 1989; **45(19)**:1721-32.
5. N.I.D.A. Annual National High School Seminar Survey. Rockville, MD, April 1993.

6. Millman RB, Beeder AB. The new psychedelic subculture: LSD, ecstasy, rave parties and the Grateful Dead. Psychiatric Ann 1994; **24(3)**:148-150.

7. Keup W. Use, indications and distribution in different countries of the stimulant and hallucinogenic amphetamine derivatives under consideration by WHO. Drug Alcohol Depend 1986; **17(2-3)**:169-92.

8. Mack RB. A bit on the Wilde side: MDMA abuse. N C Med J 1985; **142(11)**:1391.

9. Aghajanian GK, Haigler HJ. Hallucinogenic indolamines. Psychophar Comm 1975; **21**:53-60.

10. Glenn RA. Do classical hallucinogens act as 5-HT2 agonists or antagonists? Neuropsychopharmacology 1990; **3(5-4)**:509-17.

11. Harris LS. The stimulants and hallucinogens under consideration: a brief overview of their chemistry and pharmacology. Drug Alcohol Depend 1986; **17(2-3)**:107-18.

12. Rold JF. Mushroom madness. Psychoactive fungi and the risk of fatal poisoning. Postgrad Med 1986; **79(5)**:218-8.

13. Leikin JB, Krantz AJ, Sell-Kanter M, Barkin RL, Hryhorczuk DO. Clinical features and management of intoxication due to hallucinogenic drugs. Med Toxicol Adverse Drug Exp 1989; **4(5)**:324-50.

14. Nichols DE. Differences between the mechanism of action of MDMA, MBDB, and the classic hallucinogens. Identification of a new therapeutic class: entactogens. J Psychoactive Drugs. 1986; **18(4)**:305-13.

15. Levi L, Miller NR. Visual illusions associated with previous drug abuse. J Clin Neuroophthalmol 1990; **10(2)**:103-10.

16. Treatment of acute drug abuse reactions. Med Lett Drugs Ther 1987; **29(748)**:83-6.

17. Giannini AJ, Quinones RQ, Sullivan BS. Fluoxetine reverses post-lysergic acid (LSD) symptoms. J Clin Pharmacol 1988; **28**:938.

CHAPTER 12

SEDATIVE-HYPNOTICS

Originally, the sedative-hypnotics were called "tranquilizers." The name continued until the 1950's when this label was reapplied to the newly introduced benzodiazepines.

From their introduction at the beginning of the twentieth century, the sedative-hypnotics were widely used as sleeping powders, sleeping pills, induction agents in surgery, and relaxants. After the introduction of the benzodiazepines and the emergence of physicians who were educated in their use, the licit use of sedative-hypnotics declined.

Ironically, at the same time, sedative-hypnotics were beginning to be used for effects other than sedation. Their greatest application presently are as anticonvulsants, although they find minor use in the treatment of colic, whooping cough and eclampsia.

Interestingly, it is the rise of managed care medicine that may account for the resurgence of their lawful use as sedating agents. Under the pressures of managed care, many surgical procedures which were previously done on an inpatient basis in a hospital are now done in hospital outpatient surgery units and in private doctors' offices. Instead of general anesthesia, patients who require minor plastic surgery, liposuction or laser cholecystectomy are typically given a sedative-hypnotic the night before surgery and a second tablet or capsule on the morning of surgery to help provide relaxation.[1,2]

LABORATORY TESTING

The sedative-hypnotics are among the most easily tested of all drugs of abuse. Generally, testing is of urine samples. Thin layer chromatography can be used to qualitatively assay all members of this group. Quantitative analysis can be provided by radioimmunoassay (RIA) or enzyme immunoassay (EIA). If testing is done for legal reasons such as confirmation of a positive employee drug screen, or assignment of responsibility in a traffic accident or fatality, gas liquid chromatography/mass spectrometry (GC/MS) is advised.[3]

Table 12-1: Sedative-Hypnotics Available in the United States

Brand Name	Generic Name	Route of Administration
Amytal	Amobarbital	p.o., IV
Antrocal	Phenobarbital	p.o.
Arco-Lase	Phenobarbital	p.o.
Bellergal	Phenobarbital	p.o.
Butisol	Butabarbital	p.o.
Donnatal	Phenobarbital	p.o.
Doriden	Glutethimide	p.o.
Equagesic	Meprobamate	p.o.
Equanil	Meprobamate	p.o.
Fiorinal	Butalbital	p.o.
*Luminal	Phenobarbital	p.o., IV, IM
MB-Tab	Meprobamate	p.o.
Meprobamate	Meprobamate	p.o.
Meprospan	Meprobamate	p.o.
Miltown	Meprobamate	p.o.
Mudrane	Phenobarbital	p.o.
Nembutol	Pentobarbital	p.o., IV, suppos.
Noludar	Methyprylon	p.o., IV
Pentothal	Thiopenthol	p.o.
Placidyl	Ethchorvynol	p.o.
PMB - 200	Meprobamate	p.o.
PMB - 400	Meprobamate	p.o.
*Quaalude	Methaqualone	p.o.
Quadrinal	Phenobarbital	p.o.
Rexatal	Phenobarbital	p.o.
Saronil	Meprobamate	p.o.
Seconal	Secobarbital	p.o.
Solfoton	Phenobarbital	p.o.
*Sopor	Methaqualone	p.o.

* Available only through illicit sources

HISTORY

The first sedative-hypnotic was barbituric acid. It was invented in 1864 by Adolph von Baeyer in Germany. He combined malonic acid and urea to produce malonyl urea. At the end of his work day, he went to a nearby beer garden, where he joined a group of Prussian soldiers who were busily celebrating the birthday of their patron saint, St. Barbara. It is from the combination of St. Barbara's name and the word "urea" that barbituric acid was named.

Barbituric acid found an immediate use in the production of riboflavin. In 1903, a derivative, barbital, was synthesized and sold by Baeyer Laboratories as a sedative under the trade name "Veronyl." In 1912, another derivative, phenobarbital, was developed. It quickly replaced the bromides paraldehyde and chloral hydrate as the sleeping pill of choice. Its adoption by both Allied and Central Powers of World War I guaranteed its familiarity by physicians on both sides of the Atlantic. In addition to its use as a sedating and soporific agent, phenobarbital became the drug of choice in surgery. It was used to initially induce unconsciousness while gaseous agents such as ether maintained the unconscious state. In the 1940's and 1950's, a number of barbiturates were developed with a variable duration of action, providing the physician with increased specificity.

In the 1950's, a number of nonbarbituric-derived hypnotics were developed. These included ethchlorvynol, which was given the name Placidyl by Abbot Laboratories; meprobamate, sold as Miltown by Wallace Laboratories; methyprylon, sold as Noludar by Hoffman-LaRoche; and glutethimide, vended as Doriden and also produced by Hoffman-LaRoche. With the explosion in the number of different sedative-hypnotics, it was ironic that the concurrent introduction of the benzodiazepines Librium and Valium by Hoffman-LaRoche marked the end of sedative-hypnotic's dominance over the soporific and tranquilizing market.

In the 1960's, the last of the sedative-hypnotics, methaqualone, was developed by Arner-Stone as Quaalude. It was quickly adopted by the medical community as the ultimate sedating agent and sleeping pill. The street community adopted it as a spurious aphrodisiac. It was thought to increase libido, lower inhibitions and prolong sexual excitement. However, none of these claims were true. Nevertheless, many enterprising but unscrupulous physicians developed a number of sex clinics and stress clinics whose reason for existence was the high volume prescription or sale of methaqualone. The existence of these clinics became a national scandal and, literally, a federal case. As a result of the Supreme Court decision in U.S. vs. Lefkowitz, these clinics were closed and methaqualone was classified as a "DEA class I" drug.

Although glutethimide, methaqualone and methyprylon are no longer manufactured the United States, they are still manufactured in Mexico and other countries. A demand still exists for all three drugs, especially methaqualone, and this, along with a fairly porous national border, guarantees a thriving black market. Other sedative-hypnotics are available, but due to DEA regulations they are preferentially obtained by addicts through the black market. Although some researchers have attributed the passage of NAFTA (the North American Free Trade Agreement) as the cause of an increase in illicit sedative-hypnotic trafficking in the United States, a review of police records in the states bordering Mexico indicates that this is not the case.[4] (See Table 12-1.)

DEMOGRAPHICS

Sedative-hypnotics remain among the least-abused drugs in the United States, especially in the younger population. Results of a National Household survey in 1989 revealed that only 14 to 19 percent of all high school seniors and young adults had experimented at least once with sedative-hypnotics for recreational purposes.

However, in spite of their relatively low use pattern, sedative-hypnotics are still of major concern to physicians. These are the largest single cause of adverse reactions reported in the emergency room. Among the recreational drugs, they are also the single largest source of overdose deaths.[5] Fifteen percent of sedative-hypnotic overdose deaths are caused by suicide, 50 percent are caused by inadvertent overdoses, and the remaining 35 percent come from other causes, including idiosyncratic reactions. Most deaths associated with recreational use of sedative-hypnotics usually occur in combination with alcohol, opiates or benzodiazepines.[6-9]

There are generally two types of sedative-hypnotic abusers: recreational abusers and medical abusers. Recreational abusers include teenagers and young adults who abuse sedatives episodically in social settings, usually in combination with other drugs. Another subtype of recreational abuser uses barbiturates in an oral or intravenous form on a regular basis, also in combination with other drugs. Because of the violence associated with long-term sedative use, these types of abusers are usually part of an isolated subculture. They tend to be unemployed or engage in only occasional employment. This is accompanied by a high incidence of antisocial behavior including the commission of violent crimes.[10,11]

The second group of abusers is made up of people who utilize sedative-hypnotics to deal with anxiety or insomnia related to their lifestyle or intrapsychic conflicts.[12] Initially, these people obtain their sedative-hypnotics from their physicians. As tolerance develops, they usually utilize the naivete of the same physician to obtain ever-increasing dosages. If this physician does not comply, the abuser will generally go to multiple physicians and pharmacies, or use a spouse or loved one to obtain sedatives from their own physicians for spurious symptoms. In some cases, this group will also begin using sympathomimetics, such as amphetamine, to counteract early morning sedation. They will sleep under the influence of a sedative-hypnotic and get started in the morning under the influence of a sympathomimetic.[13]

PHARMACOLOGY

All of the sedative-hypnotics except for meprobamate (Equanil, Meprobamate, Saronil), work through gamma-aminobutyric acid (GABA). GABA acts to gate the chloride channels. These channels serve an inhibitory function by shutting down activity of the more stimulatory neurotransmitters such as the biogenic amines.[14] Sedative-hypnotics operate at a specific receptor, the B-P (barbiturate-pyridoxine) receptor within the GABA receptor chloride channel complex.[15] The effect of the sedative-hypnotics is very powerful and direct, unlike the benzodiazepines working at B-Z co-receptors and exerting a more indirect influence upon the chloride channels.[16] (For further discussion of the GABA-complex, see Chapter 5, Benzodiazepines.)

The most frequently used sedative-hypnotics, the barbiturates, are usually taken orally and are absorbed in the small intestines. When barbiturates are taken as sodium salts or coingested with alcoholic beverages, absorption is increased. Relative lipid solubility determines the amount of albumin binding, the degree of vascular uptake, and the time needed to achieve equilibrium. Highly lipid-soluble barbiturates are more quickly absorbed, allow equilibrium to be achieved more quickly, and are of shorter duration than are those that are less lipid-soluble. Highly lipid-soluble barbiturates are metabolized by side chain oxidation and subsequent glucuronidation, N-hydroxylation, and ring cleavage. Less lipid-soluble barbiturates are generally not metabolized and are excreted unchanged. Excretion is generally renal and increased by alkalinization.[17]

Ethchlorvynol is relatively rapid-acting. Drowsiness is achieved within 15 minutes, with peak action occurring in one hour. Duration is five hours with a half-life of 10 to 20 hours. Ethchlorvynol is metabolized by oxidation and conjugation, and is excreted renally. It is considered highly addictive. Ethchlorvynol is not recommended for prescription because the manufacture of this compound requires carbon tetrachloride, which has been implicated in the destruction of the ozone layer.[18]

Glutethimide is highly lipid soluble and has a half-life of approximately 10 hours. It is metabolized in the liver by initial hydroxylation followed by glucuronidation. It is 50 percent albumin bound and 98% metabolized. Excretion is exclusively renal.[19]

Meprobamate is generally taken orally with peak levels achieved within 1 to 3 hours. Absorption is through the small intestine. It is less than 5 percent albumin bound. It is 90 percent metabolized in the liver by hydroxylation and glucuronidation, and is excreted renally.[20]

Methaqualone is highly lipid soluble and absorbed in the small intestine. Peak levels are achieved within two hours. It is highly albumin bound with a half-life of 2 to 3 hours. It is metabolized by N-oxidation and hydroxylation. Its pharmakinetics are bicompartmental with a distribution half-life of 1 hour and an elimination half-life of 10 to 40 hours.[21]

Methyprylon is absorbed in the small intestine, although in many cases it is injected intravenously and occasionally intramuscularly. It is highly water soluble with very little lipid solubility. It is 95 percent metabolized in the liver exclusively by glucuronidation. Absorption occurs within 1 to 2 hours with peak levels achieved within 2 to 3 hours. Half-life is 4 to 5 hours and excretion is renal.[22]

Most sedative-hypnotics, especially barbiturates, methaqualone and glutethimide, tend to induce hepatic enzymes. Exceptions include ethchlorvynol and meprobamate which have little such activity. Sedative-hypnotics also tend to interact synergistically with opiates, alcohol, benzodiazepines, methadone and propoxyphene HCl. In fact, some fatalities have been unknowingly produced by the co-administration of propoxyphene HCl with short-acting or intermediate-acting barbiturates.[23,24]

MEDICAL COMPLICATIONS

The major complication of sedative-hypnotics occurs because of their hazardous interaction with alcohol, opiates, methadone, propoxyphene HCl and benzodiazepines. This interaction can produce centrally mediated respiratory arrest and centrally and peripherally mediated cardiac depression. In addition, sedative-hypnotics should never be prescribed for patients with acute intermittent porphyria or porphyria variegata, since these can increase porphyria synthesis.[25]

Overdoses of sedative-hypnotics suppress the central nervous, cardiovascular and respiratory system, and may reduce renal function. An EEG generally shows a burst-suppression pattern. In this particular pattern, there are short-lived periods of high activity followed by electrical silence. Suppression of these various symptoms produces apnea, coma, laryngospasm and hypotension leading to cardiovascular collapse. Chronic abuse of sedative-hypnotics may lead to hip fracture, especially in elderly patients.[26,27]

Sedative-hypnotic withdrawal is the most dangerous of all the withdrawals experienced in the field of drugs of abuse. Various authors have estimated a 5 to 20 percent mortality rate in nontreated subjects. Although the severity is a function of dosage and duration of the addiction, all barbiturate addicts being detoxified should be treated with caution.

At the very least, they should be placed on seizure precautions with padded bed rails. EKG monitoring should be instituted. Nearly three-fourths of patients in unassisted withdrawal will experience grand mal seizures which, in some cases, can progress to status epilepticus. Body temperatures can exceed 101°F, going as high as 103°F or higher. There is also accompanying delirium with visual misperception and visual hallucinations.[28] Many cases appear similar to that of alcohol detoxification but are much more severe. Death may occur during status epilepticus cardiac collapse, apnea, or hyperthermia.[29,30] In this latter case, the colloquial street expression, "your brain is being fried on drugs," is accurate. Patients detoxifying from barbiturates, especially in unassisted withdrawal, will have intense symptoms followed by a period of prolonged sleep. They will awaken totally detoxified if they survive.[31-33]

DIAGNOSIS

There are three types of diagnostic categories in the abuse of sedative-hypnotics. The addiction, overdose and withdrawal state all produce quite different syndromes. The addicted patient presents with many psychiatric components, including mixed anxiety and depression, which sometimes progresses to suicidal ideation. There many be panic, phobias and paranoia, which may or may not be associated with social withdrawal. Generally, there is poor hygiene and a foul breath. Memory is decreased in all three spheres. Often, poor speech formation may progress to slurring. The muscles tend to be flaccid and the patient is usually flexic or hyporeflexic. Pupils are constricted and Romberg's sign may be present. Patients who inject sedative-hypnotics tend to present with bullae.[34,35]

In overdose, the patient appears delirious, lethargic or comatose. Babinski reflex is generally present. The skin is diaphoretic, dehydrated and very cold to the touch. Body temperature is generally hypothermic; diastolic and systolic blood pressure is decreased. The pulse is thready and respiratory excursions are diminished in frequency and intensity. During early overdose pupils are constricted; in later stages, they are dilated and fixed. There is Cheyne-Stokes breathing, atelectasis, and evidence of pulmonary edema.[36] Laboratory testing reveals acidosis and uremia. EEG patterns are characterized by a burst-suppression pattern.[37]

During the withdrawal state, the patient tends to be irritable. He is disoriented and may be delirious. Nausea progressing to vertigo and emesis can also be present. Generally, there is a weakness with hyperreflexia or possibly hyporeflexia. Dysarthria and dysphagia are present. The patient is generally anxious with a progression to panic phobias. Content may be paranoid. Gross resting tremors are present and there is generalized ataxia.

As withdrawal progresses, postural hypertension increases, high fever ensues and there may be cardiac arrhythmias. At this point, the patient will complain of formications, an akathesia-like syndrome, and severe insomnia. If not properly detoxified, body temperature can exceed 103°F. Convulsions that sometimes progress to status epilepticus occur in nearly one-third of untreated patients.[38]

⅓ see p 151

TREATMENT

If the habitual dosage is unknown, the physician may determine the equivalent sedative-hypnotic dose by giving a pentobarbital test dose. Generally, 200 mg. is administered orally and the patient observed after one hour. Patients with a daily habit of less than 400 mg. of barbiturate or equivalent will be sleepy but arousable; those who chronically abuse 400 to 600 mg. will have slurred speech and nystagmus in the horizontal plane. If the addiction is in the 600 to 1000 mg. range, nystagmus but not slurred speech is present. If no symptoms are observed, the dosage equivalent is in excess of 1000 mg. of barbiturates per day.

Table 12-2: Dosage Conversion Table for Sedative-Hypnotics

Amobarbital	100 mg
Butabarbital	100 mg
Ethchlorvynol	750 mg
Glutethimide	250 mg
Meprobamate	400 mg
Methaqualone	300 mg
Methyprylon	150 mg
Pentobarbital	100 mg
Phenobarbital	30 mg
Secobarbital	100 mg

Once the daily dosage is determined by this method, the patient is given phenobarbital 30 mg. orally for each 100 mg. of pentobarbital equivalent. The dosage is reduced by 10 percent or 30 mg. of phenobarbital per day, whichever is less. If withdrawal symptoms occur, then immediately administer phenobarbital 200 mg. orally and revise the dosage schedule upward. This method may also be used if the addictive dosage is known by giving the phenobarbital equivalent.[39] (See Table 12-2.)

In cases of overdose, withdrawal hypothermia is treated with warming blankets. Hyperthermia generally responds to administration of phenobarbital or other sedative-hypnotics. Convulsions respond to administration of phenobarbital as do hallucinations and tremors.

If arrhythmias emerge, prescribe digoxin 0.5 to 0.75 mg orally as a loading dose, with digoxin 0.25 mg. every six hours until digitalization is achieved. After the patient is digitalized, digoxin is prescribed in the amount of 0.25 mg. every day as necessary.

Acidosis is treated by 80 mEq KCl per L in D5/W at a rate of 50 mEq per L. After urine flow is initiated, add bicarbonate to produce 0.45 percent isotonicity. Hypotension is treated by norepinephrine 2 ampules per 500 cc of D5/W with flow rate titrated against blood pressure. Atelectasis is treated by bronchial toilette or bronchoscopy. Other respiratory difficulties are treated by 100 percent oxygen by nasal canula. If more severe, the patient must be intubated; or a tracheotomy should be performed if necessary. Uremia is treated by hemodialysis.

If the patient presents with acute overdose, prescribe apomorphine 0.1 mg. per kg. subcutaneously to induce emesis. If the patient is overdosed on a short-acting barbiturate, lavage with 1-to-1 saline-caster oil emulsion. If the staff is not familiar with this type of emulsion, lavage with activated charcoal slurry 75 to 100 grams. To increase renal elimination of the absorbed barbiturate, hydrate with 0.45 N saline to which has been added sodium bicarbonate 100 mEq in O.45 N saline. Then inject furosemide 40 mg. intramuscularly. Furosemide injection may be repeated in 4 to 6 hours.[40]

TYPICAL CASE PRESENTATION

The patient was a 37-year-old white male who was admitted on a voluntary basis to a hospital detoxification unit. He had been abusing secobarbital at a rate of 400 to 600 mg. at bedtime for three years. On occasion, he would use his wife's butalbital when he "just couldn't sleep."

He began using secobarbital due to insomnia engendered by the stresses associated with a job promotion. As he developed tolerance, his physician compliantly increased the dosage. This physician, however, retired and the new doctor refused to continue her colleague's prescribing practices.

The patient was placed on bed rest with seizure precautions. Vital signs were ordered every hour for 24 hours. Using dosage conversion charts, he was placed on phenobarbital 30 mg. orally every 5 hours, daily. This dosage was reduced to 15 mg. the second day and by 10 percent each day thereafter. On day four, the man began manifesting gross tremors and mild confusion. He complained of nausea and vertigo. An additional dose of phenobarbital 10 mg. orally was given with good results. The withdrawal dosage was plateaued for two days and then the withdrawal schedule was re-initiated. At day eight, he was taken off bed rest and completed withdrawal without incident.

With the cooperation of his new physician, he accepted an outpatient referral to a psychiatrist for treatment of insomnia and possible depression. However, he refused referral to an outpatient drug rehabilitation center.

NOTES

1. Klein JA. Anesthesia for liposuction in dermatologic surgery. J Dermatol Surg Oncol 1988; **14(10)**:1124-32.
2. Marten TJ. Physician-administered office anesthesia. Clin Plast Surg 1991; **18(4)**:877-89.

3. Maurer HH. Identification and differentiation of barbiturates, other sedative screening procedure using computerized gas chromatography-mass spectrometry. J Chromatogr 1990; **530(2)**:307-26.

4. Giannini AJ. (Unpublished research.)

5. Pinch WJ, Dougherty CJ. Competency after a suicide attempt: an ethical reflection. Dimens Crit Care Nurs 1993; **12(4)**:206-11.

6. Ross HE. Alcohol and drug abuse in treated alcoholics: a comparison of men and women. Alcohol Clin Exp 1989; **13(6)**:810-6.

7. Lester D, Abe K. The effect of controls on sedatives and hypnotics on their use for suicide. J Clin Toxicol 1989; **27(45)**:299-303.

8. WHO Expert Committee on Drug Dependence. Twenty-fourth report. World Health Organ Tech Rep Ser 1988; **761**:1-34.

9. Lester D. Iatrogenic concerns in the treatment of suicidal patients. Pharmacol Toxicol 1991; **69(4)**:301-2.

10. Roache JD, Griffiths RR. Abuse liability of anxiolytics and sedative-hypnotics: methods assessing the likelihood of abuse. NIDA Res Monogr 1989; **92**:123-46.

11. Williams P, Bellantuono C, Fiorio R, Tansella M. Psychotropic drug use in Italy, national trends and regional differences. Psychol Med 1986; **16(4)**:841-50.

12. The treatment of insomnia. Drug Ther Bull 1990; **28(25)**:97-8.

13. Melander A. Henricson K, Stenberg P, Lowenhielm P, Malmvik J, Sternebring B, Kaij L, Bergdahl U. Anxiolytic-hypnotic drugs: relationships between prescribing, abuse and suicide. Eur J Clin Pharmacol 1991; **41(6)**:525-9.

14. Ooi R, Feldman S. The hypnotic actions of alpha 2-adrenoceptor agonists. Anaesthesia 1992; **47(10)**:909.

15. Inoue O, Kobayashi K, Suhara T. Effect of sedative drugs upon receptor binding in vivo. Prog Neuropsychopharmacol Biol Psychiatry 1992; **16(6)**:783-9.

16. Yeh HS, Dhopesh V, Maany I. Seizures during detoxification. J Gen Intern Med 1992; **7(1)**:123.

17. Miller NS, Gold MS. Sedative-hypnotics: pharmacology and use. J Fam Pract 1989; **29(6)**:665-70.

18. Greenblatt DJ, Harmatz JS, Shader RI. Clinical pharmacokinetics of anxiolytics and hypnotics in the elderly. Clin Pharmacokinet 1991; **21(3)**:165-77.

19. Morgan WW. Abuse liability of barbiturates and other sedative-hypnotics. Adv Alcohol Subst Abuse. 1990; **9(1-2)**:67-82.

20. Rickels K. The clinical use of hypnotics: indications for use and the need for a variety of hypnotics. Acta Psychiatr Scand Suppl 1986; **332**:132-41.

21. Hale WE, May FE, Moore MT, Stewart RB. Meprobamate use in the elderly. A report from the Dunedin program. Am Geriatr Soc 1988; **36(11)**:1003-5.

22. Greenblatt DJ, Harmatz, Shader RI. Clinical pharmacokinetics of anxiolytics/hypnotics: rational and laboratory lore. Br J Addic 1991; **21(3)**:165-77.

23. Busto EU, Sellers EM. Anxiolytics and sedative-hypnotics dependence. Br J Addict 1991; **86(12)**:1647-52.

24. Bergman H, Gorg S, Engelbrechtson K, Vikander B. Dependence on sedative-hypnotics: neuropsychological impairment, field dependence and clinical course in a 5-year follow-up study. Br J Addict 1989; **85(2)**:301.

25. Verstraete AJ, Bogaert MG, Buylaert WA. Placing obsolete hypnotics on prescription and the admission rate for acute poisoning with these drugs. Eur J Clin Pharm 1990; **39(5)**:519-20.

26. Templeton JS. Dependence on sedative-hypnotics. Br J Addict 1990; **85(2)**:301.

27. Daly MP. Drugs and the risk of hip fracture. J Am Geriatr Soc 1990; **38(6)**:727-8.

28. Lowenthal DT, Nadeau SE. Drug-induced dementia. South Med J 1992; **84(5 Suppl 1)**: S24-31.

29. Yeh HS, Dhopesh V, Maany I. Seizures during detoxification. J Gen Intern Med 1992; **7(1)**:123.

30. Boutroy MJ. Drug-induced apnea. Biol Neonate 1994; **65(3-4)**:252-7.

31. de Wit H, Griffiths RR. Testing the abuse liability of anxiolytic and hypnotic drugs in humans. Drug Alcohol Depend 1991; **(1)**:83-111.

32. Balter MB, Uhlenhugh EH. The beneficial and adverse effects of hypnotics. J Clin Psychiatry 1991; **52 Suppl**:16-23.

33. Miller F, Whitcup S, Sacks M, Lynch PE. Unrecognized drug dependence and withdrawal in the elderly. Drug Alcohol Depend 1985; **15(1-2)**:177-9.

34. Ballinger BR. New drugs. Hypnotics and anxiolytics. BMJ 1990; **300(6722)**:456-8.

35. Holm M. Intervention against long-term use of hypnotics/sedative in general practice. Scand J Prim Health Care 1990; **8(2)**:113-7.

36. Henson LC, Ward DS. Effects of anesthetics and sedatives on the control of breathing. Ann Acad Med Singapore 1994; **23(6 Suppl)**:125-9.

37. Caranasos G, Busby J. Sleep disorders, constipation and pain: George Caranasos and Jan Busby [interview by Richard L Peck]. Geratrics 1985; **40(8)**:87-8,90.

38. Chiang WK, Goldfrank LR. Substance withdrawal. Emerg Med Clin North Am 1990; **8(3)**:613-31.

39. Giannini AJ, Slaby AE, Giannini MD. Handbook of Overdose and Detoxification Emergencies. New Hyde Park, Medical Examination, 1992.

40. Jayner G, Galloway G, Wiehl WO. Haight-Ashbury free clinics' drug detoxification protocols—Part 3: Benzodiazepines and other sedative-hypnotics. J Psychoactive Drugs 1993; **25(4)**:331-5.

CHAPTER 13

STEROIDS

All steroids are based upon a molecular structure made up of 17 carbon atoms arranged in a four-ring structure. These carbon atoms are, in turn, bonded to 28 hydrogen atoms. Steroid molecules start with a base structure, "squalene." Additional carbon groupings produce a variety of biologically-active compounds in humans. These include riboflavin, hydrocortisone, aldosterone, cholesterol and biosteroids.

There are nearly 30 different steroid hormones, but the ones most often abused are analogues of the androgenic (male) hormone, testosterone. They are usually known as "anabolic steroids." Anabolic steroids used for purposes of abuse include natural testosterone plus synthetic derivatives (see Table 13-1).

When taken in large amounts, anabolic steroids increase body mass, muscular strength and endurance. They may be used on a regular off/on schedule of 16 weeks, then discontinued for four to eight weeks. This procedure, called "cycling," is used to avoid detection by drug testing. When steroids are taken in combination, it is called "stacking." During cycling, if the dosages are gradually increased and then decreased, it is called "pyramiding." Finally, when several drugs are taken in a pyramidal fashion, it is know as "stacking the pyramid.[1,2]

LABORATORY TESTING

The steroids are the most difficult of all the drugs of abuse to detect, since many of them are metabolized to testosterone. Steroids metabolized to testosterone esters include stanozolol, methandrostenolone, and methenolone. If they are not metabolized, they may be detected in urine samples with the use of gas chromatography or mass spectrometry. Steroids metabolized as testosterone, testosterone cypionate or testosterone enanthate are detected by ratio determination. The ratio of testosterone to epi-testosterone is usually less than 3 to 1 in a healthy individual. A ratio greater than 6 to 1 is considered a positive test for

Table 13-1: Anabolic Steroids Available in the United States

Brand Name	Generic Name	Commonly Used Route
Adroyd	Oxymetholone	p.o.
Anadrol	Oxandrolone	p.o.
Delatestryl	Oxymetholone	p.o.
Depo-testosterone	Testosterone enanthate	IM
Dianabol	Testosterone cypionate	IM
Durabolin	Methandrostenolone	p.o.
Equipoise	Nandrolone dicanoate	IM
Finaject	Boldenone	IM, s.q.
Halotestin	Bolasterone	IM, s.q.
Innovar	Fluoxymesterone	p.o.
Maxibolin	Ethylestrenol	p.o
Metandren	Methyltestosterone	p.o.
Oranebol	Oxymesterone	p.o.
Oreton	Methyltestosterone	p.o.
Primobolan	Methenolone	IM, p.o.
Testex	Testosterone propionate	IM, p.o.

anabolic steroid abuse. If the ratio is between 3 to 1 and 6 to 1, the person is usually labeled as "possibly abusing."

A number of nondiagnostic laboratory changes are seen with steroid use. There is generally increased liver function with changes in glucose. Low-density lipoprotein is increased but high-density lipoprotein is decreased, resulting in a net increase in total cholesterol levels. Hormones and peptides dependent on testosterone or estrogen functioning are altered. This means there may be a decrease in luteinizing hormone and follicle stimulating hormone but an increase in cholecystokinin. In patients using testosterone ester-based anabolic steroids, testosterone levels are increased, but for those using anabolic steroids not based on testosterone ester, there is a net decrease in serum testosterone. Sperm count may be decreased. Occasionally there is a change in sperm pathology.[3-6]

HISTORY

The first use of anabolic steroids occurred in Neolithic times when warrior hunters of Europe and Central Asia ate the raw and cooked testicles of such powerful animals as the bull and the horse. There is also some conjecture that the Aztec jaguar warriors, an elite group of fighting men, ate the testicles of their human sacrifices, especially if they were powerful warriors.

During the Medieval era, the Roman gladiators in Spain metamorphosed into an early equivalent of modern matadors. In addition to cutting the ears, tail and noses of the bull, they would also cut off the testicles, throw them on a fire to cook and then eat them. A similar practice occurred in the nineteenth century in America. After castrating a bull, American cowboys, Mexican vaqueros and Argentine gauchos cooked and ate the fresh testicles of the newly-created steers.

In the seventeenth century, the first medicinal steroid was employed: digitalis, a steroid glucoside extracted from fox blood. However, medicinal use of anabolic steroids did not begin until the twentieth century. In 1931, androsterone, a testosterone metabolite, was isolated in urine. In 1935, testosterone was isolated from testicular extracts. Later that year, testosterone was synthesized from dioxegenin.

In the late 1940's, non-anabolic steroids were used to treat crippling forms of arthritis. In the 1950's, anabolic steroids were initially used by competitive body builders and Olympic athletes. Systematic abuse was practiced by the East German and Soviet athletes, especially in those events where endurance, strength and mass were paramount. Over the years, steroids were increasingly taken by athletes in other countries as well. However, use decreased when RIA testing was introduced in the 1984 Olympics. Also that year, RIA testing revealed that approximately 20 percent of all NCAA football players in the United States abused steroids.[7]

DEMOGRAPHICS

It has been estimated that over 1 million Americans have at one time used anabolic steroids to enhance body performance or increase muscle mass. The population of steroid abusers is concentrated among athletes, body builders and weight lifters. It has been estimated that 15 to 20 percent of all body builders and weight lifters have abused steroids, and of this group, approximately 70 percent are male. Abuse, however, seems to begin in late adolescence. Approximately 500,000 to 700,000 high school students have abused steroids at some time. Approximately 4 to 10 percent of all boys and up to 2.5 percent of girls used steroids. This percentage increased dramatically among male college athletes. Approximately 20 percent have been reported to use steroids in this group. In raw numbers, this translates into approximately 200,000 NCAA athletes per year. Reasons given for steroid use among young adults include "bulking" (i.e., increasing muscle mass), prolonged endurance, increased strength, and overall improvement of performance.[8-11]

Most steroids are acquired through legal sources. The majority come from China, Germany, or other European countries where medical practice differs from that in the U.S. In some cases, however, athletes have been able to obtain steroids from physicians who disagree with the prohibition of steroids. Also, steroids are stolen from various physicians and veterinary offices. Currently, there is no evidence of large-scale illegal production of steroids in the United States.[12,13]

PHARMACOLOGY

Anabolic steroids vary in structure, route of administration, duration of action, and relative toxicity. All anabolic steroids can be classified into three groups: testosterone, 17-α-alkylated steroids, and 17-ester steroids. Because oral testosterone is oxidized in the liver after ingestion, it is generally given intramuscularly. Esterification or alkylation, however, protects against oxidation of the 17-β-hydroxy moiety during the first pass through the liver. As a result, the 17-α-alkylated steroids and the 17-ester steroids can be taken either intramuscularly or by oral administration. The apparent advantage of these two groups is offset by the very real risk of hepatic toxicity.

Testosterone is readily absorbed after oral dosing but has poor bioavailability due to the above mentioned first-pass effect. Only 50 percent reaches circulation. Orally administered methyl-testosterone is less extensively metabolized and has a longer half-life. Injectable steroids require infrequent administration. They are designed as depot drugs and are released slowly from the injection site. Although they are metabolized more quickly in the liver than are oral steroids, they need to be injected only at 14 to 30-day intervals. Half-lives of the depot-injectable steroids are as long as a week.[14]

Intracellularly, steroids stimulate the growth of muscle cells during normal development. Steroids do not increase the *amount* of actual muscle cells. Receptor binding at specific steroid receptors in the nucleus increases RNA production, which results in an increased rate of protein synthesis.[15,16] Activity at calcium channels, tyrosine kinase, and G-6-P-D enzyme may increase activity level and endurance. This may be synergized by anti-GABA activity.[17-19] Anabolic "growth" effects and androgenic (i.e., "masculinizing") effects are caused by different receptor effects at different tissues and not, as mistakenly believed, by differential effects of different types of steroids. Actually, steroids tend to have very little specificity because the anabolic-responsive muscle cells have the same receptors as androgen-target cells. As a result, all anabolic steroids have androgenic activity and can produce masculinizing effects, especially in female abusers.[20]

MEDICAL COMPLICATIONS

Major complications of steroid use focus on the blood pressure and liver. Sustained use of steroids can cause a chronic increase in blood pressure with acute exacerbation leading to the possibility of cerebral vascular accidents and myocardial infarctions.[21] Also, in the manner of a positive feedback loop, anabolic steroids can produce liver damage, which is associated with a decreased rate of metabolism and decreased rate of synthesis of those very plasma proteins responsible for steroid binding.[22] As a result, repetitive use increases levels of free steroids in the plasma. There is a saturation of receptor sites and thus an increased rate of hepatic toxicity.[23] In addition to hepatic toxicity, anabolic steroids are associated with hepatic and possibly other site tumor formation.[24]

Other major effects include an increased incidence of noncancerous masses and cancer. There is also diminished immunity for both bacterial, viral and fungal infections. A minor effect is a distinctive rash consisting of raised, reddish or occasionally tan rubbery elements throughout the face and body.[25] Adolescents and preadolescents can experience premature epiphyseal closure, while adults may have osteonecrosis.[26] Children may develop virilization or feminization, and in males, there may be pronounced gynecomastia. Epiphyseal closure as well as some hypothesized "molding" effects in younger abusers may produce a permanent alteration in physique and proportion. Occasionally, chronic steroid use can result in glaucoma.[27]

Psychiatric effects include depression of suicidal proportions, mania with large mood swings, aggressiveness with violent behavior, and frank psychosis. The patient may become dangerous to those around him, including health care providers. If psychosis or aggressiveness progresses, physicians and other members of the team are advised to proceed with caution. Occasionally, the pendulum of the patient's mood may swing back, creating severe depression or catatonia.[28]

DIAGNOSIS

It is difficult to misdiagnose the typical steroid abuser. If steroid abuse has occurred for many years and is associated with weight lifting, the person will be quite large in size. The shoulders, chest, arms and legs create a "hulking" appearance. A steroid rash and cushingoid appearance will support the diagnosis.

Male addicts tend to have testicular atrophy and will complain of impotence or sterility. They will have enlarged breast tissue and scalp hair loss proceeding to baldness. They may complain of dysuria or occasional constipation due to enlargement of the prostate. Elsewhere hirsutism may be produced. There are complaints in both sexes of diminished libido as well as hyperphagia.

Women generally complain of amenorrhea, increased clitoral size and diminished breast size. We have also observed previously unreported remolding and possible increased density in the mandibles of female patients, but not of male patients.

Generally, addicts tend to be labile with alterations between suicidal depression and increased aggressiveness. Psychosis is generally of paranoid, persecutory ideation. Manic phases seldom involve grandiosity.[29]

The withdrawal state is associated with suicidal depression, insomnia, anorexia, cravings for steroids, extreme fatigue, akathisia, and occasionally formications. Visual hallucinations are also seen. Many steroid addicts perceive a white chromatopsia which persists during the withdrawal phase and may indeed intensify. This chromatopsia is experienced as a general "bleaching" of color in the environment.[30]

TREATMENT

Currently, no "magic bullet" exists for treating steroid abusers that acts as clonidine acts for opiate addicts or bromocriptine for cocaine addicts. Detoxification therefore requires specific pharmacological intervention. Medical intervention is supportive and symptomatic.

Depression is best treated with fast-acting antidepressants such as the serotonergic reuptake inhibitors. Prozac 80 to 100 mg. orally, daily or

Effexor 225 to 425 mg. daily have been found to be effective. Headaches and musculoskeletal pains are best treated by the nonsteroidal anti-inflammatory drugs (NSAIDs). Severe lability can be treated with carbamazepine 200 mg. two to three times a day, or valproic acid in variable doses. Anxiety and tremors can be treated by benzodiazepines or hydroxyzine. If no depression is present, symptoms of anxiety as well as tremors can be easily treated with beta-blockers such as propranolol 10 to 30 mg. three to four times a day.

Hypogonadism can be treated with appropriate hormonal replacement dependent upon the patient's sex. Extreme caution must be used, however, since the sexual hormones are in themselves powerful steroids. They may induce steroidal cravings in an otherwise recovering steroid addict.

The steroidal rash can be quite disfiguring. Unfortunately, there is no known treatment. Make-up can be used to cover a facial rash. Although controversial, some physicians have recommended tattooing. However, these tattoos are large and may not be acceptable to many patients.

It has been observed that denial or rationalization are among the highest in this group of drug abusers. Steroids do not ordinarily produce intoxication. Many steroid addicts deny that they have addiction. They justify the beneficial effects, including enhanced performance and increased muscle mass, while ignoring the pathological symptoms. Much tension is generated in the detoxification unit, since steroid abusers do not identify with other addicts. As a result, we have observed a structure in which steroid addicts avoid other addicts and use their increased muscle mass to aggressively obtain isolation as well as defend themselves against any hostility thus engendered.

Because of the personality and motivation of the typical steroid addict, rigorous physical therapy is absolutely essential in the inpatient program. However, for some addicts weight training equipment may act as a visual trigger and could cause a relapse and withdrawal cravings. In treating steroid abusers, care must be taken to patiently explain that the patient's strength, mass and endurance will all decrease. Thus the steroid addict will experience a decrease in size, strength and performance while other nonsteroidal addicts will become relatively more fit. This can also lead to tension and may interfere or sabotage the rehabilitation phase. The treatment team must endeavor to help these types of addicts find acceptable alternative sources of self-esteem while dealing with a loss of power and autonomy.

see p 207 "art of 6 months"

TYPICAL CASE PRESENTATION

The patient was a 22-year-old, white female who presented for evaluation to the drug-treatment unit psychiatrist. She reported a four-year history of abusing steroids, including "stacking" and "pyramiding" practices. She explained that she began going to the gym because she was tired of being little. "I started lifting but nothing was happening so they started selling me Dianabol and it started working. Then I started taking more." The patient continued to abuse steroids until her source was arrested. After a two-week frantic but fruitless search for another source, she decided to seek detoxification.

The patient complained of severe depression lasting throughout the day, anergia and insomnia. There was also amenorrhea, diminished libido and constriction headaches. She was quite anxious, irritable and admitted to "punching out a couple of women." This hyper-irritability had been present for the past year.

Physical examination revealed an extremely well-developed, anxious, white female. Vital sings were remarkable for tachycardia. Gross resting tremors were present. Hirsutism was noted. The patient had a number of large tattoos which were obtained "to cover up all the bumps." Below the tatoo ink was noted a pink, raised rash. The raised areas were rounded or flat, and rubbery to touch. Mental status examination was remarkable for dysphoria, irritability and lability.

She was admitted to the inpatient treatment unit. Since the patient had already discontinued the steroids, the decision was made not to titrate downward. Depression was treated with venlafaxine which was titrated upwards to 225 mg. daily. Anxiety was treated with oral hydroxyzine 50 mg. one to three times a day as needed. Headaches were treated with acetaminophen 500 mg. up to three times a day. On the fifth day, the patient became extremely labile and threatening to female staff members and other patients. With her permission, she was placed on carbamazepine 100 mg. three times a day which quickly reduced this behavior.

While on the unit, the patient tended to be generally aloof. She could not relate to other patients because she felt she was not a drug addict. She remained alone until a male steroid addict was admitted to the unit. The two quickly formed an exclusive dyad and refused to participate in group activities, though they did interact in individual therapeutic modalities. When informed that this behavior was unacceptable, they both signed out against medical advice. The patient, however, did agree to enter an outpatient rehabilitation program "just so I can get my medication." She was then given discharge instructions. She was advised not to enter into a sexual relationship with the other steroid addict. She was reminded that she should expect her body size and strength to decline as muscle-mass decreased in size. Finally, she was advised to avoid exercise spas and weight rooms because these environments could trigger a re-addiction to steroids.

NOTES

1. Giannini AJ, Miller NS, Kocjan DK. Treating steroid abuse: a pediatric perspective. Clin Pediatrics. 1991; **30(9)**:538-542.
2. Hall PF. The role of endozepine in the regulation of steroid synthesis. Mol Neurobiol 1995; **10(1)**:1-17.
3. Dandidiker WB, DeSaussare VA. Fluorescence polization in immunochemistry. Immunochem 1970; **7**:799-828.
4. White JH, McCuaig KA, Mader S. A simple and sensitive high-throughput assay for steroid agonists and antagonists. Biotechnology 1994; **12(10)**:1003-7.
5. Nunez EA, Haourigui M, Martin ME, Benassayag C. Fatty acid and steroid hormone action. Prostaglandins Leukot Essent Fatty Acids 1995; **52(2-3)**:185-90.
6. Jausons-Loffreda N, Balaguer P, Roux S, Fuentes M, Pons M, Nicholas JC, Gelmini S, Pazzagli M. Chimeric receptors as a tool for luminescent measurement of biological activities of steroid hormones. J Biolumin Chemilum 1994; **9(3)**:217-21.
7. Becchi M, Alguilera R, Farizon Y, Flament MM, Casabianca H, James P. Gas chromatography/combustion/isotope-ratio mass spectrometry analysis of urinary steroids to detect misuse of testosterone in sport. Rapid Commun Mass Spectrum 1994; **8(4)**:304-8.
8. Buckley WE, Yesalis CE, Fried K, et al. Estimated prevalence of anabolic steroid use among male high school seniors. JAMA 1988; **260**:3441-5.
9. Dezelsky TL, Toohey JV, Shaw RS. Non-medical drug use behavior at five United States universities: a 15 year study. Bull Narc 1985; **37**:49-53.
10. Bergman R, Leach RE. The use and abuse of anabolic steroids in Olympics-caliber athletes. Clin Ortho Related Res 1985; **198**:169-72.

11. Johnston LD, O'Malley PM, Bachman JG. 5th Annual National Survey of American High School Seniors. University of Michigan News and Information Services. Ann Arbor, Michigan 1990.

12. Boudreau F, Konzak B. Ben Johnson and the use of steroids in sport: sociological and ethical considerations. Can J Sport Sci 1991; **16(2)**:88-98.

13. Zhou J. Bioactive glycosides from Chinese medicines. Mem Inst Oswaldo Cruz 1991; **86(Suppl 2)**:231-4.

14. Baulieu EE. Neurosteroids: an overview. Adv Biochem Psychopharmacol 1992; **47**:1-6.

15. Smith RG, Nag A, Syms AL, et al. Steroid receptor, gene structure and molecular biology. J Steroid Biochem 1986; **214**:51.

16. Lebrethon MC, Jaillard C, Naville D, Bégeot M, Saez JM. Regulation of corticotropic and steroidogenic enzyme mRNAs in human fetal adrenal cells by corticotropin, angiotensin-II and transforming growth factor beta 1. Mol Cell Endocrinol 1994; **106(1-2)**:137-43.

17. Mendoza C, Soler A, Tesarik J. Nongenomic steroid action: independent targeting of a plasma membrane calcium channel and a tyrosine kinase. Biochem Biophys Res Common 1995; **210(2)**:518-23.

18. Gordon G, Mackow MC, Levy HR. On the mechanism of interaction of steroids with human glucose 6-phosphate dehydrogenase. Arch Biochem Biophys 1995; **318(1)**:25-9.

19. Nguyen Q, Sapp DW, Van Ness PC, Olsen RW. Modulation of GABAA receptor binding in human brain by neuroactive steroids: species and brain regional differences. Synapse 1995; **19(2)**:77-87.

20. Danzo BJ, Joseph DR. Structure-function relationships of rat androgen-binding protein/human sex hormone binding globulin: the effect of mutagenesis on steroid-binding parameters. Endocrinology 1994; **135(1)**:157-67.

21. Mochizuki RH, Richter KJ. Cardiomyopathy and cerebrovascular accident associated with anabolic-androgenic steroid use. Physician Sports Med 1988; **16**:109-14.

22. Ishak KG, Zimmerman HJ. Hepatotoxic effects of the anabolic/androgenic steroids. Semin Liver Dis 1987; **7**:230-6.

23. Nowakowski H. Metabolic studies with anabolic steroids. Acta Endocrin. 1962; **63(Suppl)**:37.

24. Creach TM, Rubin A, Evans DJ. Hepatic tumors induced by anabolic steroids in an athlete. J Clin Pathol 1988; **41**:441-3.
25. Lobo RA. Investigating the cause of hirsutism and acne in women. Clin Chem 1995; **41(1)**:12-3.
26. Usher BW, Friedman RJ. Steroid-induced osteonecrosis of the humeral head. Orthopedics 1995; **18(1)**:47-51.
27. Chong NH. Glaucoma induced by steroids. BMJ 1994; **309(6950)**:343.
28. Fink M. Steroid-induced catatonia. BR J Psychiatry 1991; **159**:445.
29. Brower KJ, Blow FC, Beresford TP, et al. Anabolic-androgenic steroid dependence. J Clin Psychiatry 1989; **50**:31.3.
30. Giannini AJ, Mahar PJ. An unusual ocular complication of thioridazine. Int J Psychiatry Med 1980; **10**:217-219.

CHAPTER 14

VOLATILE SUBSTANCES

The volatiles constitute a class of psychoactive substances whose delivery system is their evaporative process. Most of these substances have industrial or domestic application and are widely available on a legal and commercial basis. They constitute a disparate group which includes aerosols, gasoline, glues, lacquer, lighter fluid, moth balls, paint thinner, room deodorizers, commercial spot removers and typewriter correction fluid. Antifreeze and degreasers, as well as substances which utilize benzene or toluene as a solvent, are also abused.

Solvents are the most toxic of all the drugs of abuse and can cause irreversible damage to the brain and liver. All volatiles share the quality of evaporation near room temperatures. This assures a short-acting intoxication effect with a rapid onset. All produce depressant and euphoric effects similar but more intense than alcohol, and can produce an acute syndrome characterized by attention and concentration difficulties, amnesia, poor judgement and an acute psychosis.[1,2]

LABORATORY TESTING

Aliphatic Hydrocarbons

Generally, routine laboratory testing is sufficient to detect the presence of aliphatic hydrocarbons whether use is chronic or acute. In acute use, arterial blood gases or headspace samples will reveal diminished oxygen concentration.[3] In patients with associated aspiration pneumonitis, there is a low complete blood count (CBC) and hematuria. Chronic use of aliphatic hydrocarbons by any route is associated with urinary cellular sediment. However, false positives can be generated by frequent use of over-the-counter analgesics such as aspirin, acetaminophen and ibuprofen.

Albuminuria is also seen with chronic as well as acute use. In tests of cerebral spinal fluid, there is increased concentration of albumin and decreased concentration of taurine. The concentration of taurine is directly related to the amount of duration of solvent exposure and, as such, provides information as to the history of abuse.[4,5]

Chest x-rays are not particularly useful even in cases of early aspiration pneumonitis, although chlorinated hydrocarbons are somewhat radiopaque. Chest x-rays, however, will show edema and other findings associated with aspiration.

Aromatic Hydrocarbons

Urine phenol levels are directly correlated with the amount of aspiration and respiratory exposure. It is noted, however, that over-the-counter medications which contain phenol may give false positives or false elevations of urinary phenol. Examples of such medications include Chloroseptic®, Pepto Bismol®, Campho-phenique®, Cepastat®, Ambisol® liquid antiseptic, Ambisol® gel antiseptic and Winthrop® swab and gargle solution. Urine phenol levels are generally less than 10 mg. per liter in nonexposed individuals. As exposure increases to 0.1 ppm, urine phenol levels climb to between 10 and 30 mg. per liter. After exposure increases to 25 ppm, urine phenol levels are in the average range of 175 to 200 mg. per liter.

Phenylmercapturic acid and T-muconic acid urine concentration are specific markers for benzene inhalation or ingestion on a chronic basis. Specific benzene levels can be measured by gas chromatography through solvent extraction. Inorganic total sulfate ratio in urine samples, however, can also be used as an indirect measure to indicate occupational exposure.

HISTORY

The first recorded use of volatile agents in Western civilization was in the *Gilgamesh Epic*. Gilgamesh encountered a man who received messages from the gods through emanations from volcanic vents.

A similar gift of the gods was granted to the oracles of Delphi, who sat above a volcanic vent that generated carbon dioxide. Because of the hypoxia, the oracle would enter into a trance-like state in which she would utter her prophecies. After many generations, when the vent was no longer functional, enterprising oracles began generating their own fumes by burning laurel leaves in a copper calyx.

During the Medieval era, Arabian chemists discovered the distillation process, making available naturally volatile solvents. According to some scholars, these solvents were sometimes employed by dervishes and warriors during the period of hegemonic Islamic civilization.

Europeans, however, did not adopt volatiles until the late nineteenth century. Nitrous oxide and other inhalant anesthetics were mass-produced for the operating theater and also legitimately produced as an entertainment novelty. Originally, it was used in upper middle-class European and American homes. Here an avant-garde host or hostess would supply the guests with nitrous oxide. This "laughing gas" was passed from person to person so that the euphoriant effects could be shared by all members of this Victorian era drug party. Nitrous oxide and other gases such as ether were also used at bordellos in the United States, the United Kingdom, France, Germany and Italy. Further spreading their use was of a decrease in price associated with increased production, making these gases more available to working class adults and even young adolescents in the amusement parks of America and Europe.

Petroleum distillates became mass-produced after the introduction of the automobile's internal combustion engine. The needs of the engine, as well as the opportunity for privacy afforded by the automobile's interior, provided a convenient enclosed space for America's "fast set" to sniff gasoline-soaked rags. In England, automobile racing enthusiasts would inhale fumes generated by pouring camphor on red-hot pieces of scrap iron.

With the increase of marijuana, alcohol and cocaine abuse during the Jazz Age (1916-1930), the popularity of nitrous oxide and distillates declined. Gasoline sniffing, however, continued through the 1930's, although it declined during the rationing of World War II. Also during the 1930's, the Depression-era movies of Fred Astaire and Busby Berkeley popularized the seltzer bottle. This provided obtainable compressed carbon dioxide cartridges or "charges." These gas cartridges put sparkle in both the cocktails and the cocktail drinkers of the Art Deco era. However, because of the large amounts of carbon dioxide available in concentrated form, carbon dioxide-induced hypoxic deaths were reported.

After Charles Revson popularized matching nail polish and lipstick, acetone, a constituent of both nail polish and nail polish remover, became available for abuse.

By the 1950's, the "model hobby" craze provided an increasing variety of volatile agents to adolescents and adults. The plastic glues provided acetone and toluene. Model-paint lacquers were sources of toluene, naphtha, methylene, methanol and benzene. Rubber cement, another hobby product, was a source of acetone, hexane, isopropanol, styrene, toluene and xylene.

With the advent of the technology to manufacture nitrogenated inert gases, whipped cream, whipped cheese, and other aerosol food products for food and for abuse. By the 1960's, spray paint had become not only a source of graffiti but also of drug abuse. Toluene and chlorinated aliphatic paint was sprayed in plastic bags and inhaled by the user in much the same way that the nitrogenated gases of aerosol cans and whipped cream were abused. This was termed "huffing" or "bagging."

During the 1970's, amyl nitrite, a medicinal aid in coronary artery disease, and isobutyl nitrite, a foul-smelling industrial solvent, began being used by men as a source for a "perfect" erection. In the 1980's, Liquid Paper® correction fluid, containing trichlorethylene, became such a commonly abused product that many companies found it necessary to store this office supply in locked cabinets.

POPULATIONS AT RISK

The profile of a typical solvent abuser is a male, 16 years of age or younger. He is generally Native American or Hispanic and is a poor student. His family is usually impoverished, dysfunctional and living in an isolated community. The typical abuser will most often use chlorinated aliphatic hydrocarbons, aromatic hydrocarbons, or toluene.[6,7]

Generally, male abusers outnumber females at a rate of two to one. The initial age of abuse is usually about 11, and usage diminishes as age increases. In surveys of high school seniors, less than 1 percent of black and white students used volatiles on a daily basis, but 10 to 13 percent had experimented at least once with some kind of volatile agent. When Native American populations were examined, it was found that over 90 percent of both sexes had experimented with volatiles, and 10 percent continued to abuse them on a daily basis. Among Hispanics, a different study found that 13 to 22 percent utilized some type of volatile on a regular or semi-regular basis.[8-11]

PHYSIOLOGY/CHEMISTRY

General

The volatile agents have widely different sources and different effects on various organ systems within the body. However, they share many attributes. All of these agents are effective through inhalation or sniffing. The high is achieved in seconds and usually produces disinhibition, euphoria, enhanced hyperactivity and perceived enhancement of sexual drive and performance. All of these agents are potentially fatal. Death usually arises from cardiac arrhythmia or, less frequently, laryngospasm and central suppression of the gag reflex.[12]

The addiction syndrome involves the dopaminergic reward centers of the teleomesencephalic system (see Chapter 6, Cocaine, and Chapter 8, Marijuana). Addiction occurs in 5 percent of abusers, usually after three to six months. A generalized withdrawal complex is associated with symptoms of anxiety, cramping, delirium, fine resting tremor, insomnia, irritability and seizures.

All volatile agents tend to exhibit cross-tolerance with each other and have a similar intoxication pattern. In the first stage, there is a feeling of grandiosity, euphoria, excitement, lightheadedness, auditory hallucinations, nausea, vomiting and frontal and prefrontal headaches. Continued use of volatile agents can produce confusion, disinhibition, delusions of vulnerability, impulsivity and severe lightheadedness.[12] In the second stage, prefrontal headaches persist and increase in intensity. These can be accompanied by tinnitus, diplopia, blurred vision, photosensitivity, conjunctivitis, rhinitis and protracted coughing.

The third stage features diarrhea, emesis, arthralgia, myalgia and angina-like pain over the precordium. In the final stage, there is dysarthria, hyperreflexia, diminished coordination, involuntary enuresis, loss of sphincter tone and convulsions. This phase may end in cardiac or respiratory arrest, which are generally fatal.[13]

Alcohols

(For a discussion of ethanol, see Chapter 2, Alcohol.)

Methanol is the most abused of the inhaled alcohols. It has both central and hepatic effects as does its metabolite, formaldehyde. Formaldehyde, in turn, is metabolized in the liver to become formic acid.

Direct effects of methanol include abdominal cramping, projectile emesis, vertigo, nausea and a generalized weakness. Acute formaldehyde formation causes retinal edema. With chronic use of methanol and subsequent in vivo production of formaldehyde, the edematous retina eventually produces permanent blindness. Methanol's end product, formic acid, produces a hemorrhagic destruction of the caudate and putamen.

Aliphatic Hydrocarbons[14,15]

The aliphatic hydrocarbons include aliphatic nitrites, gasoline and n-hexane. The aliphatic nitrates constitute a grouping of extremely volatile and highly flammable liquids. Unlike most volatiles, the aliphatic nitrites have medicinal value. They are used in the treatment of angina pectoris, cyanide poisoning and hydrogen sulfate poisoning, and as a diagnostic tool for testing ventricular septal defects.

The most commonly abused forms of aliphatic nitrites are amyl nitrite and isobutyl nitrite. Both are potent, smooth-muscle relaxers which produce arterial dilation. This relaxation is nonspecific and not dependent upon adrenergic, cholinergic or serotonergic innervation. The aliphatic nitrites, however, can be antagonized by any drug that is a muscle activator. In this manner, nitrites act as functional antagonists to acetylcholine, histamine, norepinephrine or serotonin by overcoming compensatory sympathetic activity. It is theorized by some investigators that the aliphatic nitrites act at a "nitrite receptor" or pseudoreceptor.[16]

Nitrites are rapidly metabolized in the liver and very little of the active nitrite reaches the systemic circulation. De-nitration takes place within the glutathione-organic nitrate reductase system in the liver, which is the rate-limiting step. Tolerance develops rapidly, usually within three to four days.[13,17]

Gasoline is found throughout the world. It is a mixture of C-4 through C-12 hydrocarbons and small amounts of naphthalenes, olefins, paraffins and some aromatics. Gasoline tends to block oxygen as well as to destroy neural tissue.

In some countries, there is also the possibility of secondary lead intoxication from the abuse of leaded gasoline. When the lead intake exceeds 0.6 mg. per day, chronic intoxication may occur, though symptoms may take several months to appear. Lead is generally absorbed and distributed in the soft tissue, primarily the liver and the kidneys. Over time, redistribution takes place in the bones, neural system, teeth and hair where is it stored and then released. Lead affects the peripheral nerves as well as the central nervous system. In addition to the effects from the hydrocarbons, the lead may produce encephalopathy, followed by an excited delirium and peripheral neuropathy, progressively increasing the number of nerves affected.[17,18,19]

N-hexane is a volatile agent found in hobby glues. Hexane can produce giddiness. Its primary site of action is at the peripheral nerves. Hexane acts by thinning the myelin and causing axonal swelling. Chronic use produces an increase in the number of axonal neurofilaments. Its major metabolite, hexane-dione, is a ketone. This active metabolite produces effects and toxicity similar to that of n-hexane.[20,21]

Aromatic Hydrocarbons

Aromatic hydrocarbons include benzene, naphthalene and toluene.

Benzene is a solvent for plastics, lacquers, resins, varnish, some paints and some types of wax. It is a lipophilic substance which is distributed to lipid sites in the bone marrow as well as in the brain. Elimination occurs through the lungs and kidneys. Metabolic degradation is by glucoronidation and sulfanation in the liver. Benzene and its metabolites act at the subcellular level. These substances bind to bone marrow-DNA to inhibit DNA and RNA synthesis, producing chromosomal aberrations.[22]

Naphthalene is eliminated through the lungs and kidneys although the elimination through exhalation is not as great as that of benzene. Metabolism takes place through dehydrogenation and sulfanation. It produces a number of equally toxic metabolites.

Toluene is a lipid-soluble aromatic which is stored in fat tissue and bone marrow. Twenty percent is eliminated through the lungs and the remainder through the kidneys. Metabolic degradation is usually through oxidation to form benzoic acid. Benzoic acid then conjugates with glycine to form hippuric acid. Its use is associated with hypophosphatemia, hypokalemia and increased levels of creatine phosphokinase.[23-25] It acts directly on nervous tissue as well as the myelin.

Halogenated Hydrocarbons

This group of hydrocarbons includes the fluorinated, chlorinated, dechlorinated and trichlorinated hydrocarbons. All of these increase cardiac cellular receptor sensitivity to catecholamines. They are therefore associated with arrhythmias. In addition, the chlorinated hydrocarbons are metabolized hepatically to form carbon monoxide.[26-28]

Glycols

Glycols are ingested and rarely inhaled, although accidental inhalation may occur. Because of its sweet flavor similar to that of Karo® syrup, ethylene glycol, a major constituent of antifreeze, may be inadvertently ingested. The glycols are metabolized in the liver and in the kidneys to form oxalate, though some metabolism may occur in the lungs. This latter route can be associated with pulmonary edema.[29]

Nitrous Oxide

Nitrous oxide is an inert gas which achieves its psychotropic effects by asphyxia. Since it is heavier than air, inhalations must be more active than the other volatile agents. It is not metabolized, it does not combine with hemoglobin, and it is carried in the plasma in solution only. Most of it is excreted unchanged through the lungs, although trace amounts diffuse through the skin.[30-32]

DIAGNOSIS

Aliphatic Hydrocarbons

The major complications are dependent upon the route of introduction. Ingestion produces emesis and diarrhea with abdominal cramping and pain. Moderate to large amounts, or prolonged exposure, can produce renal tubular damage. In many cases, all but the most viscous of these hydrocarbons can induce aspiration. Ingestion is also associated with central nervous system depression followed by excitation.

Complications of aspiration include aspiration pneumonitis, hypoxia, pulmonary edema, cyanosis, hemoptysis, tachypnea, and pneumatocele.[33]

Inhalation can produce respiratory effects including pulmonary edema, aspiration pneumonitis, cyanosis, pneumatocele, hemoptysis and tachypnea. In addition, inhalation is associated with a high level of ventricular tachycardia and ventricular arrhythmias. Neurological complications are the same as ingestion.[34]

Rarely, aliphatic hydrocarbons are injected. In addition to all of the above mentioned complications, users who favor this route experience fever which may exceed 102° F. At the injection site, localized muscular swelling and edema develop, which usually progresses to localized muscle necrosis.[35]

Aromatic Hydrocarbons

Medical complications of aromatic hydrocarbon exposure are much more dramatic than those of the aliphatic hydrocarbons. Acute dermal or inhalation exposure can produce vascular congestion, cutaneous burns, pulmonary edema and alveolar hemorrhage. Acute dermal exposure can also produce arrythmia, edema or blistering.

Both chronic and acute exposure can result in cardiac arrhythmia as well as chronic bronchial irritation, hoarseness or cough. Occasionally, chronic exposure is associated with pulmonary edema. Neurologically, there is progressive euphoria, headaches, giddiness, vertigo and ataxia. Long-term exposure, or short-term exposure to high levels of aromatics, can produce confusion, seizure and coma. Low-level exposure can produce anorexia, dizziness, fatigue and headaches. Gastrointestinal effects are generally produced by ingestion only. These include subjective burning sensations in all oral mucosae. When this occurs in the esophagus and the stomach, it produces cramping and emesis. Hepatotoxicity can occur through all forms of exposure of both acute and chronic duration.

COMPLICATIONS

Aromatic Hydrocarbons

Generally, patients who abuse volatiles share certain symptoms. These include dizziness, fatigue, euphoria and intestinal complaints. In many cases there is cyanosis. Inhaled forms generally produce symptoms associated with the eye, including photosensitivity, photophobia, areflexia and blurring of vision. These are due to retinal edema.

Aliphatic hydrocarbons generally have a high degree of urinary cellular sediment and urinary albumin than other volatile forms.

The aromatic hydrocarbons as a group produce generalized symptoms. Specific members, however, can have certain distinctive effects. Benzene is associated with skin erythema or blistering. Toluene can produce rhabdomyolysis and projectile vomiting, cataracts, retinal tears and retinal hemorrhaging. Styrene has no special effects but naphthalene abusers tend to retain the characteristic "moth ball" odor in the breath. Naphthalene acutely can produce a profound diaphoresis associated with severe emesis. Chronic xylene abuse is associated with corneal damage and hemorrhagic pulmonary edema. Ketones tend to produce peripheral numbness and an associated overall feeling of well-being.[36]

The nitrites are associated with cyanosis and sustained penile erection. Gasoline produces intense visual hallucinations associated with ataxia and clonus.

TREATMENT

Aliphatic Hydrocarbons

Initial treatment consists of administering 100 percent humidified supplemental oxygen to assist in ventilation. Exposed skin and eyes should be well flushed with water. If breathing difficulties persist, the patient should be intubated and should receive ventilation support. Decreased serum hemoglobin should be treated with a transfusion of packed red blood cells. Mechanical ventilation should be continued as long as necessary. (Cases have been documented of mechanical ventilation being required for six or more weeks.) Much of the treatment of aliphatics is similar to that of aromatic hydrocarbons.[37,38]

Aromatic Hydrocarbons

When the patient presents, the priority should be given to protection of the airway and to seizure control. Alert patients should be placed in the Trendelenburg or left-lateral decubitus position. Suction should be instituted if necessary. Airway protection is secured in the unconscious patient by cuffed endotracheal intubation.

Seizures can be controlled by intravenous use of diazepam. The adult dose is 5 to 10 mg. intravenously over a two to three minute interval. Repeat every 10 to 15 minutes to a maximum of 30 mg. In children aged 3 days to 5 years old, the dosage is 0.2 to 0.4 mg. per kg. to a maximum of 5 mg. This maximum is raised to 10 mg. in children over 10 years of age. If circumstances prevent the use of an intravenous line, lorazepam may be given at low doses intramuscularly. Cases of rectal introduction of diazepam have been published, but this lacks FDA approval.

If seizures do not respond to diazepam, administer phenytoin by slow IV push at a rate of less than 0.5 mg. per kg. per min. (i.e., 50 mg. per min.). The initial loading dose of phenytoin in adults is 15 to 18 mg. per kg. The adult maintenance dose is 100 mg. orally or intravenously every 6 to 8 hours, maintaining a serum concentration of 10 to 20 µg. per ml. The pediatric loading dose is 15 to 20 mg. per kg. (i.e., 250 mg. per square meter of phenytoin). The IV administration rate should not be in excess of 0.5 to 1.5 mg. per kg. per min. The pediatric maintenance dose is 1.5 mg. per kg. every 30 minutes to a maximum daily dose of 20 mg. per kg. In all cases, administer the phenytoin under EKG and blood pressure monitoring. The infusion should be stopped if either arrhythmia or hypertension develops. After each injection of phenytoin, inject sterile saline through the same needle.[39]

If the physician is not familiar with phenytoin use, phenobarbital may be used. The loading dose of phenobarbital in adults is 600 to 1200 mg. diluted in 60 cc of 0.9 saline. This solution is given at a rate of 20 to 50 mg. per min. In administering an adult maintenance dose of phenobarbital, the dosage range is 120 mg. to 240 mg. every 20 minutes. In children, the phenobarbital loading dose is 15 to 20 mg. per kg. at a rate of 25 to 50 mg. per min. In children, the dosage of phenobarbital is 5 to 10 mg. per kg. every 20 minutes. No maximum dosage has been established for either adult or children.[16]

Because of the risk of seizures as well as respiratory depression, emesis is not recommended. Instead, gastric lavage may be performed with a 36-42 French tube in adults or a 24-32 French tube in children. Activated charcoal may be slowly administered in aqueous saline or sorbitol mixtures. The dosage is 30 grams of charcoal per 240 ml. of diluent. The usual dosage is 32 to 100 grams in adults, 15 to 30 grams in children, and 1 to 2 grams per kg. in infants. Both saline and sorbitol act as cathartics and should not be administered to those patients with ileus. In addition, saline catharsis should not be administered to patients with impaired renal function. Repetitive use of sorbitol or saline catharsis is not recommended.

When using non-saline cathartics without charcoal, provide a dose of 20 to 30 grams of magnesium sulfate or 4 ml. per kg. of magnesium citrate to a maximum of 300 ml. per dose. In children, this should be reduced to 250 mg. per kg. per dose of magnesium sulfate or 4 ml. per kg. per dose of magnesium citrate up to a maximum of 300 ml. per dose. If sorbitol is preferred it can be administered at a rate of 1 to 2 grams per kg. per dose to a maximum of 150 grams per dose. In children this is reduced to 1 to 1.5 grams per kg. per dose at a 35 percent solution. It is given at a maximum of 50 gm. per dose in children over 1 year. Sorbitol is not recommended in infants.[24]

Skin and eye exposure should be treated with large amounts of water. Persistent pain, swelling or lacrimation should be referred to an ophthalmologist familiar with aromatic poisoning. EKG monitoring is mandatory. Arrhythmias and other EKG changes can result directly from the aromatic solvent poisoning or secondarily from the gastric lavage.[40] Use of epinephrine is not recommended because of myocardial hypersensitization.[41]

TYPICAL CASE PRESENTATION

Because of the large number of different types of volatiles, no "typical" case can be presented.

NOTES

1. Chadwick O, Anderson R, Bland M, Ramsey J. Neuropsychological consequences of volatile substance abuse: a population based study of secondary school pupils. BMJ 1989; **298(6689)**:1679-83.
2. Dunmont MP. Psychotoxicology: the return of the mad hatter. Soc Sci Med 1989; **29(9)**:1077-82.
3. Streete PJ, Ruprah M, Ramsey JD, Flanagan RJ. Detection and identification of volatile substances by headspace capillary gas chromatography to aid the diagnosis of acute poisoning. Analyst 1992; **117(7)**:1111-27.

4. Li YM, Brostedt P, Hjertèn S, Nyberg F, Dilberring J. Capillary liquid chromatography-fast atom bombardment mass spectrometry using a high-resolving cation exchanger, based on a continuous chromatographic matris. Application to studies on neuropeptide peptidases. J Chromatogr B Biomed Appl 1995; **664(2)**:426-30.

5. Chao TC, Lo DS, Koh J, Ting TC, Quek LM, Koh TH, Koh-Tan CY, Subaidah A. Glue sniffing deaths in Singapore: volatile aromatic hydrocarbons in post-mortem blood by headspace gas chromatography. Med Sci Law 1993; **33(3)**:253-60.

6. Rojas LM, Salamanca-Gomez F. Psychological study in children addicted to inhalation of volatile substances. Rev Invest Clin 1989; **41(4)**:361-5.

7. Coulehan JL, Hirschl JW, Brillman J, et al. Gasoline sniffing and lead toxicity in Navajo adolescents. Pediatrics 1983; **71**:113-117.

8. Ostrow DG, Deltran ED, Joseph JG, DiFranceisco W, Welch J, Chmiel JS. Recreational drugs and sexual behavior in the Chicago MACS/CCS cohort of homosexually active men. Chicago Multicenter AIDS Cohort Study (MACS)/Coping and Change Study. J Subst Abuse 1993; **5(4)**:311-25.

9. Esmail A, Meyer L, Pottier A, Wright S. Deaths from volatile substance abuse in those under 18 years: results from a national epidemiological study. Arch Dis Child 1993; **69(3)**:356-60.

10. Inhalant use. N.I.D.A. Notes **2**:20-21 (1988/1989).

11. Inhalant Date in D.A.W.N. Rockville, Maryland, N.I.D.A., Div. Epidemiol. June 1988.

12. Linen CH. Volatile substances of abuse. Emerg Med Clin North Am 1990; **8(3)**:559-78.

13. Bradberry SM, Whittington RM, Parry DA, Vale JA. Fatal methemoglobinemia due to inhalation of isobutyl nitrite. J Clin Toxicol 1994; **32(2)**:179-84.

14. Couri D, Nachtman JP. Toxicology of alcohols, ketones and esters: inhalation. In: CW Sharp, Brehm ML (Eds.), Review of inhalants: euphoria to dysfunction. U.S. Government Printing Office, Washington DC, 1977.

15. Edeh J. Volatile substance abuse in relation to alcohol and illicit drugs: psychosocial perspectives. Hum Toxicol 1989; **8(4)**:307-12.

16. Flanagan RJ, Ruprah M, Meredith TJ, Ramsey JD. An introduction to the clinical toxicology of volatile substances. Drug Saf 1990; **5(5)**:359-83.

17. Chadwick OF, Anderson HR. Neuropsychological consequences of volatile substance abuse: a review. Hum Toxicol 1989; **8(4)**:307-12.

18. Burns CB, Powers JR, Currie BJ. Elevated serum creatine kinase (CK-MM) in petrol sniffers using leaded or unleaded fuel. J Clin Toxicol 1994; **32(5)**:527-39.

19. Faucett RL, Jensen RA. Addiction to the inhalation of gasoline fumes in a child. J Pediatr 1952; **41**:364.

20. Janse P, Richter LM, Griesel RD. Glue sniffing: a comparison study of sniffers and non-sniffers. J Adolesc 1992; **15(1)**:29-37.

21. Von Oettingen WF. The toxicity and dangers of aliphatic and aromatic hydrocarbons. Yale J Biol Med **15**:167-184.

22. Troutman WG. Additional deaths associated with the intentional inhalation of typewriter correction fluid. Vet Hum Toxicol 1988; **30(2)**:130-2.

23. Winek GL, Collom WD, Wecht CH. Fatal benzene exposure to glue-sniffing. Lancet 1967; **1**:683.

24. Streicher HZ, Gabor PA, Moss AH et al. Syndromes of toluene sniffing in adults. Ann Intern Med 1981; **94**:758-762.

25. King MD, Day RE, Oliver JS, et al. Solvent encephalopathy from toluene inhalation. Br Med J 1981; **283**:663-665.

26. Brady WJ, Stremski E, Eljaiek L, Aufderheide TP. Freon inhalational abuse presenting with ventricular fibrillation. Am J Emerg Med 1994; **12(5)**:533-6.

27. Fitzgerald RL, Fishel CE, Bush LL. Fatality due to recreational use of chlorodifluoromethane and chloropentafluoroethane. J Forensic Sci 1993; **38(2)**:477-83.

28. Rojas LM, Salamanca-Gomez F. Psychological study in children addicted to inhalation of volatile substances. Rev Invest Clin 1989; **41(4)**:361-5.

29. Bart-Goggs JRC, Rovini FX, Herrington TS. Glycol inhalation: diagnosis and treatment. J Royal Soc Med. 1995: **1**:874-875.

30. Pollard TG. Relative addiction potential of major centrally-active drugs and drug classes: inhalants and anesthetics. Adv Alcohol Subst Abuse 1990; **9(1-2)**:149-65.

31. Layzer RB. Myeloneuropathy after prolonged exposure to nitrous oxide. Lancet 1978; **2**:1227-1230.

32. Eckenhuff JE, Helrich M. The effects of narcotics, thiopental and nitrous oxide upon respiration. Anesthesiology 1958; **19**:240-253.

33. Johns A. Volatile solvent abuse and 963 deaths. Br J Addict 1991; **86(9)**:1053-6.
34. Miller NS, Gold MS. Organic solvent and aerosol abuse. Am Fam Physician 1991; **44(1)**:183-9.
35. Flanagan RJ, Ives RJ. Volatile substance abuse. Bull Narc 1994; **46(2)**:49-78.
36. Saker EG, Eskew AE, Panter JW. Stability of toluene in blood: its forensic relevance. J Anal Toxicol 1991; **15(5)**:246-9.
37. Shepard RT. Mechanism of sudden death associated with volatile substance abuse. Hum Toxicol 1989; **8(4)**:287-91.
38. Schwartz RH, Peary P. Abuse of isobutyl nitrite inhalation (Rush) by adolescents. Clin Pediatr 1986; **25(6)**:308-10.
39. Swadi H. Neurophysiological consequences of volatile substance abuse. BMJ 1989; **299(6696)**:458-9.
40. Nee PA, Llewellyn T, Pritty PE. Successful out-of-hospital defibrillation for ventricular fibrillation complicating solvent abuse. Arch Emerg Med 1990; **7(3)**:220-3.
41. Caputo RA. Volatile substance misuse in children and youth: a consideration of theories. Int J Addict 1993; **28(10)**:1015-32.

CHAPTER 15

EATING DISORDERS: ADDICTION BY ANOTHER NAME

Eating disorders may be considered as but another type of drug abuse. If drug abuse can be considered as behavior that: acts as a primary drive superseding other behaviors, occupies a great deal of the subject's attention, depletes resources with risk to the body's health, and destroys social, sexual and occupational relationships; then the eating disorders are indeed a form of drug abuse.

The drive for the consumption of food is, by definition, a primary drive. In the eating disorders, the need to consume food or to avoid it occupies a great deal of the individual's time and psychological effort. The medical consequences and cost of large amounts of food, laxatives etc. are expensive. As a result of obesity or unnatural thinness, health suffers, sexual desire and the number of available sexual partners is reduced, social relationships become estranged, and job performance declines.[1]

There are three types of eating disorders: obesity, the over-consumption of food; anorexia, the act of voluntary starvation; and bulimia, the voluntary purging of over-consumed amounts of food. The eating disorders derive from a multifactorial etiology making diagnosis and treatment very difficult and frustrating. Because of social and intrapsychic demands, many patients have transformed the simple act of eating into a sometimes tragic, always painful and occasionally deadly practice.[2]

HISTORY

Obesity has been a component of Western culture since the days of prehistory. Paleolithic statuaries such as the Lundendorff Venus, a statuette on display in the Berlin Museum, portray thoroughly obese bodies. Obesity continued into classical times. During the fifth century B.C., the great sculptor Polycleitus theorized perfect human dimensions using mathematical ratios. Usually, however, the reaction against obesity was expressed aesthetically, rather than mathematically.

Bulimia was first noted in Xenophon's *Anabasis*, a journal of Greek soldiers retreating through the mountains of what is present-day Turkey. Anorexia and bulimia were also practiced in the cult of Adis and Cybele. In this cult's supreme sacrament, the men castrated themselves after a period of prolonged starvation.[3] During the Roman phase of classical antiquity, bulimia became a socially accepted practice. At great and small banquets, wealthy and middle-class citizens would consume 20 or more courses and then be escorted to a small room near the dining area called a vomitorium. This room was equipped with fountains, scented flowers and water. Here the Roman guests would purge themselves of previous courses, and slaves would clean their faces and clothing so that they could return to the feast and engorge themselves anew.[4]

During the early Middle Ages, the necessity of survival precluded the emergence of many eating disorders.[5] The frequent man-made and natural depredations mitigated against obesity, not to mention anorexia and bulimia. Starvation was the most frequent nutritional disorder. However, as Europe moved into the middle and high Gothic periods, with a more stable social order and general prosperity, forced emesis again emerged.[5] Both anorexia and bulimia were used by religious penitents to ritualistically purge themselves of their sins while sometimes producing "visions." Monks practiced anorexia to sharpen their wit and reduce sexual desire. Medical professors, pharmacists and barbers prescribed powerful emetics, sometimes on a chronic basis. This ascetic view towards the human body continued into the early Renaissance.[6]

The Christian ideal was then married to the resurgent Greco-Roman ideal of the "perfect mind in a perfect body." During this period, men and women were encouraged to be slim and supple. The paintings of contemporary Renaissance artists such as Giovanni Pisano's "Madonna" and Sandro Botticelli's "Venus" depicted women with lithe, graceful and boyish appearances. The humanistic tones emerging from Renaissance Florence spread through Italy and later all of Europe. Pressure to maintain a slim body was reinforced among men through the fashion of long hose, short breeches, open shirts and slashed doublet.

During this time, anorexia and bulimia appeared among both young and middle-aged adults, especially males, due to sartorial, intellectual and social pressures. Both Renaissance papal diarist and chancellor, Johannes Burchard, and Florentine educator, Marsilio Ficino, recorded the use of purgatives and starvation diets.[7]

In the Baroque period, both men and women became gradually more obese. We can trace this through the works of the late Renaissance painters such as the elderly Titian (Tiziano Vecelli), Peter Paul Rubens and his contemporaries. This trend towards obesity continued until the end of the Napoleonic Wars. In the years following Waterloo, a general prosperity ensured that all but the very poor could afford to eat meat in abundance. To accompany the meat, Western European society developed high-caloric sauces, savories and gravies.[8]

It was at this time, however, that physicians began to associate obesity with some medical disorders.[9] They began to advise their patients to eat less. Their reduction diets for 3000 to 5000 calories per day may seem excessive to us, but were considered Spartan by their nonmedical contemporaries. The doctors' diets invariably advised white meats, vegetables and whole grains. Gradually, the upper class began to exercise and produced the "talented amateurs" who participated in the first modern Olympic games. Obesity began to emerge as a disease of the lower classes, whose diet emphasized starch and red meat.[10]

A social dichotomy emerged: the rich and upper-middle class began to suffer from anorexia and bulimia, while the lower and lower-middle classes became progressively more obese. As work itself became less labor-intensive, the upper classes began to exercise more, consuming their caloric excess, while the lower classes abjured exercise as work they didn't get paid for.[11]

DEMOGRAPHICS

The eating disorders share many demographic characteristics with classical drug abuse. In examinations of populations with anorexia and/or bulimia, up to 20 percent of these patients are shown to abuse alcohol or other drugs. When the opposite situation is examined, 2 to 12 percent of all drug abusers report symptoms consistent with anorexia, whereas 5 to 25 percent report bulimia. Another 15 percent meet current definitions of obesity, which include individuals whose body fat makes up greater than 25 percent of their total body weight for men, and greater than 30 percent of their total body weight for women.[12,13]

One recent, large-scale study demonstrated that 50 percent of all female bulimics were reported to have alcoholic relatives.[14] Other studies have shown that nearly 20 percent of bulimics had alcoholic or drug abuse disorders in their first- or second-degree relatives. Our own studies in progress show that 50 percent of all female anorectics have alcoholic or drug abusing first- and second-degree relatives, whereas 25 percent of all female bulimics and 20 percent of all male bulimics have alcoholic or drug abusing relatives.

Though anorectics and bulimics are usually female, there is a 15 percent incidence of anorexia among the elderly, divided equally among both sexes.

PHARMACOLOGY

General feeding behaviors are regulated by the hypothalamus. Satiety is controlled by the ventral-medial center. Feeding and hunger are under the control of the lateral center.

As discussed in Chapter 1, Medical Bases of Addiction and Withdrawal, the neurotransmitters that are the mediators for drug addiction are the same as those involved in eating disorders. Serotonin, which is acted on by psychedelics and phencyclidine, also acts upon the satiety center. Norepinephrine, which effects both the satiety and the feeding centers, is also implicated in sympathomimetic abuse. Dopamine, a major neurotransmitter in cocaine abuse and possibly alcoholism, acts upon the feeding center. Opioids tend to act in concert with dopamine on the feeding center.

The major effect of serotonin is stimulation of the satiety center at the $5HT_{1B}$ receptor, causing a decrease in feeding behavior. The minor effect of serotonin is inhibition of satiety centers at the $5HT_{1A}$ receptors causing a mild increase in feeding behavior. In addition, some activity at the feeding center is inhibited at both $5HT_{1B}$ and $5HT_{1A}$ centers. The overall effect of these contradictory actions is to decrease feeding behavior. Serotonergic activity, in fact, is so powerful that it can override noradrenergic, dopaminergic and opioid activity, at least at the satiety center.

Unlike serotonergic activity which affects feeding behavior, norepinephrine acts mainly to increase meal size, especially carbohydrate intake. Noradrenergic activity at both the satiety and feeding centers is exerted through the α_2-receptor. There also seems to be synergistic interaction with dopamine. Dopamine activity at the feeding center is a function of its concentration. At low levels it increases feeding behavior, but at higher levels it decreases feeding behavior. Norepinephrine also inhibits corticotropic releasing factor (CRF), which acts to reduce food intact. Thus, norepinephrine works directly by its activity on feeding and satiety centers and indirectly by CRF inhibition.

Like norepinephrine, opioids help modulate feeding behavior through associative dopaminergic activity. The majority of opioid activity is exerted on the feeding center at the κ-receptor upon which dynorphin acts. There is, however, some activity at μ- and Δ-receptors. Opioids tend to increase cravings for fatty and savory foods. Opioid activity is mediated by zinc. Independent of opioid activity, zinc deficiencies directly tend to diminish the ability to taste sweet or salty foods. In addition, the opioid peptide cholecystokinin (CCK) lowers serum cholesterol levels, diminishes opioid-induced gastrointestinal analgesia, increases anxiety levels and reduces appetite. High levels of cholesterol, however, will reverse the anti-analgesic effects of CCK.

Anorexia

Many biochemical models have been hypothesized to explain anorexia. Some lines of research have focused on the role of the neurotransmitter "substance P." This transmitter relates complex taste information from the taste buds to the central nervous system via the paraventricular nucleus in the hypothalamus. In many elderly anorectics but in only a few young anorectics, there is a reduction in the amount of available substance P.[15]

Some studies have also noted decreases in CRF production, dynorphin levels and zinc levels in anoretics. Zinc activity is noted to decline with age and in people experiencing severe physical or emotional stress. This may account for the development of a forme-fruste anorexia in marathon runners and triatheletes.[2]

It has been hypothesized that in some anoretics, the hypothalamic-pituitary-adrenal axis has been destabilized. This is thought to be due to disruption of noradrenergic over-regulation of CRF release from the hypothalamus. The dexamethasone depression test (DST) provides similar results in depressed patients, cushingoid patients, euthymic anorectic patients, and steroid addicts.

The activity of norepinephrine and CRF may also be affected by the opioids. CRF, which is in itself a powerful anorexigenic agent, can assist in the breakup of β-lipotropin to form the opioid, β-endorphin. In opiate addiction, such drugs as morphine replace β-endorphin as a natural ligand. Morphine then acts upon opioid receptors in the locus coeruleus to inhibit norepinephrine release. Morphine addiction is associated with anorectic symptoms. Abrupt morphine withdrawal produces symptoms which may be alleviated by a high intake of sugar or a simple carbohydrate. Complete relief can be obtained by using the presynaptic α-2-agonist, clonidine, to down-regulate a noradrenergic release. Chronic use of clonidine, however, can produce depression and anorectic symptoms.[16]

The resemblance between anorexia and the effects of drug abuse does not extend only to opiates. The emphasis on body shape, size and extreme physical activity that is exhibited in those suffering from eating disorders is behaviorally similar to the activity of steroid abusers.

Bulimia

In contrast to the multifactorial etiology in anorexia, many researchers have described bulimia as a hyperserotonergic state. As a result of increased levels of serotonergic activity, the patient experiences diminished satiety.

Fenfluramine, a known anorectic agent, produces increased serotonergic release as well as reuptake inhibition. Several blind studies have shown that treatment with fenfluramine reduces binging behavior and voluntary emesis. Generally, fenfluramine action produces diminished food intake within several hours and diminished emesis within 24 hours.[15]

Sixty mg. of the serotonergic reuptake inhibitor fluoxetine can give comparable results.[17,18] The use of predominantly noradrenergic antidepressants such as desipramine and maprotiline reduce binging behavior but have indeterminate effects upon voluntary emesis. Clinical trials with naltrexone and naloxone, a weak κ-antagonist, have produced essentially mixed results.

Neuropeptide-Y, a polypeptide, may also play a role. When cerebral spinal fluid samples of bulimic women were examined, it was found that neuropeptide-Y levels were elevated. However, post-treatment bulimics, as well as anorectics and controls, had normal levels of neuropeptide-Y. Our own unpublished studies have shown a relationship between low levels of the serotonergic metabolite 5HIAA and increased levels of neuropeptide-Y in the cerebral spinal fluid of recovering bulimics.

Obesity

Obesity seems to be an inherited genetic disorder based upon the involvement of multiple genetic factors. It has long been known that local administration of any of the catecholamines at the medial hypothalamus causes a short-term increase in food intake. A surgical vagotomy below the level of the diaphragm, however, reduces the level of intake. Because of the effects on the vagus by these biogenic amines, catecholamine as well as indolamine etiologies have been hypothesized.

Increased serotonergic activity or decreased noradrenergic activity can increase carbohydrate craving. A drop in central dopamine levels in the lateral hypothalamus can reduce protein consumption whereas decreased opioid activity in this area can increase cravings for fatty or savory foods. A number of case reports and open studies of the effects of cocaine upon appetite have implicated dopamine in cravings for salty as well as fatty foods.[19]

Whereas the opioids increase overall feeding, activity at other receptors produces different results. Activity of µ- and κ-receptors reduces food intake; κ- and Δ-activity promotes expenditure of body energy; and ε-peripheral receptors promote energy conservation.

The dopaminergic responses in alcoholism, cocaine and amphetamine addiction on the one hand, and obesity on the other, show similarities. Since dopaminergic activity may stimulate the reward system, it may be that excess dietary intake is a response to diminished central dopamine activity. High alcohol intake is associated with down-regulation of the dopamine DA-2 post synaptic receptor. Receptor sensitivity furthermore increases during the early phases of withdrawal. Growth hormone secretion is under dopaminergic influence. Growth hormone release is similarly influenced in obesity and alcoholics. The sympathomimetics amphetamine and cocaine are also associated with disordered dopaminergic regulation.

MEDICAL COMPLICATIONS

Anorexia

Anorexia shares the effect of balanced starvation. Body temperatures of less than 36.3°C (97.3°F) are noted in nearly all anorectic patients, and cardiovascular instability is often seen. Postural hypotension with decreases in systolic blood pressure greater than 20 mm. Hg are frequently noticed. EKG changes include abnormal T-wave morphology, ST segment depression and bradycardia with nodal escape. AV block, atrial fibrillation, flutter, ventricular ectopy, escape, tachycardia and sinus arrest are also seen.

Amenorrhea or menstrual irregularity is found in post-pubescent female anorectics. Usually there are low levels of luteinizing hormone (LH) and follicle stimulating hormone (FSH) which respond to weight gain. Male sexual hormones seem to be relatively unaffected in anorexia although some researchers have reported low testosterone levels. There is usually a diminished thyroid stimulating hormone (TSH) response to thyroid releasing hormone (TRH) challenge, as well as low T3 and T4 serum levels.

Renal electrolyte effects of anorexia are generally related to either dehydration or water loading. There may be elevated or decreased BUN according to the amount of hydration. Overall, hypokalemia, but not hypochloremia, is common. A CBC-Diff usually reveals leukopenia with relative lymphocytosis, anemia, and occasionally thrombocytopenia associated with bone marrow hypoplasia. As a result of long-term starvation, patients develop constipation, delayed gastric emptying, superior mesenteric artery syndrome, and gastric dilatation.

Bulimia

The induced emesis, laxative abuse, and diuretic abuse practiced by bulimics can result in severe electrolyte imbalances. Hypokalemia, hypochloremia and metabolic alkalosis are commonly observed. Hypocalcemia and hyponatremia are also occasionally seen. When combined with semi-starvation, these electrolyte imbalances and alkalosis can produce EKG changes which are similar to (although usually more severe than) those seen in anorectic patients.

EKG abnormalities include atrial fibrillation, atrial flutter, bradycardia, first degree AV block, second degree AV block, intraventricular conduction disturbance, right bundle branch block, ventricular escape, ventricular tachycardia and, occasionally, ventricular fibrillation. There has also been demonstrated impairment of left ventricular contractility and pericardial effusion. Some bulimic patients with anorexia develop congestive heart failure if the weight gain recovery phase is too rapid.

Hormonal disturbances of bulimia mirror those of anorexia except that elevated cholecystokinin levels may be seen in the latter condition. Gastrointestinal responses are also similar, except that bulimia may cause bilateral parotid enlargement. This is commonly viewed as a hypertrophic response to chronic irritation by gastric hydrochloric acid. Esophagitis, esophageal ruptures, esophageal varices and, occasionally, pancreatitis may be seen. Dental caries result from the effects of gastric acid and enzymes upon tooth enamel and gum.

Obesity

Obesity tends to be associated developmentally with a earlier onset of puberty. In obese children, there is increased incidence of slipped femoral epiphyses and tibia vara. Both children and adults can be somnolent and drowsy due to the elevated concentration of carbon dioxide levels found in what is called pickwickian syndrome. Hypertension and an increased incidence of myocardial disease are seen in obese patients. There is also increased incidence of orthopaedic abnormalities and diabetes mellitus.

DIAGNOSIS

Anorectics are usually characterized as men and women who have an overwhelming fear of weight gain or obesity. This fear persists even when they are quite thin; their bodily distortion forces them to see themselves as obese. This distortion, however, does not extend to others and they are able to accurately identify thin, obese and underweight individuals. They tend to over-emphasize their body weight or body shape, and deny any medical problems related to their induced starvation. Their body weight is generally less than 85 percent normal weight for their height and age. In adolescent, adult, and premenopausal adult women, there is amenorrhea for at least three consecutive cycles.

Bulimic patients engage in episodes of binge eating. During relatively short intervals, extraordinarily large amounts of food are consumed. Nearly all bulimics feel themselves to be out of control during these episodes.

Binge-eating episodes are often followed by compensatory episodes to prevent weight gain. These behaviors include self-induced emesis, misuse of diuretics, misuse of laxatives, misuse of enemas, or injections of insulin. Some bulimics as well as anorectics may exercise excessively. These excessive activity periods are characterized by more than 60 minutes of weight lifting activity or more than 2 hours of aerobic activity *in direct response* to a period of binging. As a result of the bulimic's excessive concern with bodily proportions and weight, the binging/purging/over-exercising period occurs at least twice weekly.

Obesity is somewhat more difficult to diagnose. Excess body mass relative to height is a convenient index. Unfortunately, it can give erroneous conclusions when applied to weight lifters who are typically heavier and possess a greater lean muscle to fat body ratio than obese people. Obesity, then, is correctly defined as a function of excess body fat. Skin-fold thickness measurements of the biceps, triceps, subscapular and suprailiac areas provide an excellent measure of fat distribution and can be used to diagnose amount of body fat. In America, men whose body fat exceeds 25 percent of the recommended weight, and women whose body fat exceeds 30 percent, are defined as obese. The ratio between the abdomen and the widest part of the buttocks is the abdominal-gluteal ratio (AGR). If it is greater than 0.8 in women and 0.9 in men, this is consistent for male pattern obesity. Men and women who meet other criteria for obesity but have a low AGR ratio are said to possess female-pattern obesity. Most obese patients provide a history of eating practices such as binging, night eating, nocturnal snacking, and continuous eating or picking behavior.

TREATMENT

Eating disorders may arise in association with drug addiction.[20,21] When eating disorders accompany other addictive behaviors, the eating disorder can be treated as an element of polydrug abuse. They share characteristics of addictive and self-destructive behavior, and treatment requires the same thing: abstinence. However, total abstinence cannot be applied to food. Rather, the approach should be to reduce pathological eating behaviors and, through peer pressure and other forms of behavioral therapy utilized in an addiction unit, gradually reshape the patient's eating habits, to become nutritional and nonpathological.[22] Dual-track programs for treating eating disorders and alcohol or drug disorders have been attempted without much success. Other researchers have made the addictive behavior a major focus and the eating disorder a minor focus.[23]

Although this has produced a somewhat positive outcome, it serves to sequester and isolate the drug abuser with an eating disorder.

Our experience has show that rather than fractioning staff resources, the eating behavior can be included within the entire spectrum of addictive behavior. In this manner, it can be included in staff conferences and group and community therapy sessions as a form of dependency. For units wishing to treat this type of patient, the triad of Alcoholic Anonymous, Narcotics Anonymous and Cocaine Anonymous can be expanded to include Overeaters Anonymous. By including the eating disorders as an element without major or minor focus, neither the drug-seeking component nor the abnormal food-intake component will be excluded to the detriment to the other.

As a thoroughly integrated element, eating disorders respond to the behavioral and cognitive techniques used in the drug and alcohol addiction programs. The goal-oriented changes in attitudes and behavior, and acceptance of the commitment to recovery are shared initial goals. As in the AA model, the patient admits his helplessness and need for a higher power. As for all other addictive behaviors, family programs attempt to include "significant others" into the healing process. Family members are educated to recognize and reduce enabling behavior as in other co-addictions. The processes of denial, intellectualization, minimization, and rationalization are addressed and disposed of within the context of the therapeutic milieu. In long-term therapy, patients are generally referred to Overeaters Anonymous *as well as* attendance at AA, NA, or CA programs.

It is to be emphasized that an eating disorder is to be treated as addictive behavior only when it accompanies drug or alcohol dependency. Neither intellectual constructs nor reported studies have demonstrated any rationale for this approach in the presence of an isolated eating disorder.

NOTES

1. Huebner HU. Endorphins, Eating Disorders and Other Addictive Behaviors, NY:WW Norton, 1993.
2. Giannini AJ, Slaby AE. The Eating Disorders. NY, Springer-Verlag, 1993.
3. Cumont F. Oriental Religions in Roman Paganism. Chicago: University of Chicago Press, 1911.

4. Gatteschi G. Restauri della Roma Imperiale. Rome: Nicolà Zanichelli Editori, 1924.
5. Hulme EM. The Middle Ages. NY: MacMillan, 1938.
6. Giannini AJ. Anorexia nervosa — a retrospective view. Int J Psychiatry Med 1981; **12(3)**:199-203.
7. Pottinger G. The Court of the Medici. London: Croom-Helm, 1974.
8. Johnson P. The Birth of the Modern. New York: Harper Collins, 1991.
9. Campbell M. The Life and Times of Sidney Owenson. London: Mercer, 1988.
10. Field M. Memoirs of Dr. Samuel Parr. London: Williams, 1828.
11. Camrie JD (Ed.). Selected works of Thomas Sydenham. London: Oxford Press, 1922.
12. Pickens RW, Heston LL. Psychiatric Factors in Drug Abuse. NY: Grune & Stratton, 1974.
13. Lacey JH, Morreli E. Bulimic alcoholics. Br J Addict 1986; **81**:38-393.
14. Pyle RL, Mitchell, Eckett ED, Halvorsen PA, Newman PA, Goff GM. This incidence of bulimia in freshman students. Int J Eating Disord 1993; **2**:75-85.
15. Giannini AJ. Drug abuse and depression. Possible models for geriatric anorexia. Neurobiol Aging 1988; **9(1)**:26-27.
16. Giannini AJ, Pascarzi GA, Loiselle RH, Price WA, Giannini MC. Comparison of clonidine and lithium in the treatment of mania. Am J Psychiatry 1986; **143**:1608-1609.
17. Russell AG, Checkley SA, Perez EL, Feldman J, Eisler J. A controlled trial of d-fenfluramine in bulimia nervosa. Clin Neuropharmacol 1988; **11**:S149-S154.
18. Enas GG, Popa HG, Vevine LR. Fluoxetine in bulimia nervosa (Abst). Presented at the American Psychiatric Association, San Francisco, May 11, 1989.
19. Dettling M, Heinz A, Dufeu P, Rommelspacher, H. Grafo KJ, Schmidt LG. Dopaminergic responsivity in alcoholism. Am J Psychiatry 1995; **152**:1317-1321.
20. Giannini AJ. Drug abuse and depression: catecholamine depletion suggested as biological tie between cocaine withdrawal and depression. Natl Inst Drug Abuse Notes. 1987; **2a(2)**:5, 1987.
21. Scott DW. Alcohol and food abuse: some comparisons. Br J Addic 1983; **78**:339-344.

22. Brisnan J, Diegal M. Bulimia and alcoholism. J Substance Abuse Treatment 1984; **1**:113-118.
23. Sweben JE. Eating disorders and substance abuse. J Psychoactive Drugs. 1987; **19**:181-182.

CHAPTER 16

CARDIOVASCULAR COMPLICATIONS OF DRUG ABUSE

With the rise in illicit drug use in the United States and worldwide, the medical community has become increasingly aware of adverse cardiovascular effects associated with drug abuse. Cardiovascular complications may manifest themselves not only in chronic offenders but also in an acute situation. Chronic abusers develop "cardiovascular tolerance" to increasing doses of the same offending agents. In novice users without such "tolerance buildup," cardiovascular complications may manifest at much lower doses.

Cardiovascular complications seen with drug abuse include myocardial infarction, cardiac arrhythmia, myocarditis and cardiomyopathy. This chapter will focus on the serious cardiovascular complications, arising from both acute and chronic use of the various agents. It is based on our experience in managing cardiovascular complications during withdrawal.

COCAINE

Since 1990, cocaine has become the third most commonly used drug, behind only alcohol and marijuana.[1] Cocaine is taken into the body through several routes. Worldwide, the most common mode of absorbing this drug is through intranasal insufflation. With continued use of the drug, many users advance to smoking and intravenous use.

Cocaine hydrochloride is a water-soluble powder that varies greatly in purity and is frequently diluted with procaine. This mixture is usually taken intravenously, but it can be smoked as well.

The use of cocaine can produce severe cardiovascular toxicity. The major cardiovascular complications of this drug are similar to those experienced in amphetamine use. Side effects include cardiac arrhythmias, myocardial ischemia and infarction, high output congestive heart failure, dilated cardiomyopathy and myocarditis. Patients with known coronary disease run a higher risk of cardiac toxicity with cocaine use. Patients with no demonstrable cardiovascular disease and with normal coronary arteries, however, can also experience cardiovascular complications from cocaine use.

In 1989, Isner et al., outlined the mechanism by which cocaine can lead to myocardial ischemia and infarction.[2] Cocaine potentiates the physiologic response to catecholamines. This action is produced by inhibition of noradrenergic receptors at storage sites in adrenergic neurons, as well as by potentiation of tyramine-facilitated norepinephrine release from these storage sites. This free-catecholamine response accelerates the pulse and raises blood pressure, thereby increasing oxygen demand. Under normal conditions, increased oxygen demand results in dilated coronary arteries. When cocaine is used, it exerts a direct vasoconstrictive effect on vascular smooth muscle. Thus, vasoconstriction occurs despite the increase in oxygen demand.[3]

This set of events, superimposed on stenotic lesions, can lead to myocardial ischemia, injury or infarction. Endothelial injury induced by vasoconstriction can lead to formation of thrombi and may cause some delayed adverse cardiovascular effects. Long-term use of cocaine may induce myocarditis or dilated cardiomyopathy in the absence of an acute event.[4]

When patients appear with acute symptoms, our approach is in many ways similar to that of all patients presenting with acute ischemic disease. These patients require careful cardiac monitoring and appropriate cardiovascular and respiratory support. It is our recommendation that they be placed in a cardiac unit, or at least in an intermediate care setting.

As previously discussed, the excess of free catecholamines is the nidus of cardiovascular complications. This problem must be addressed supportively and pharmacologically. Beta-blocking agents which block both the α- and β-adrenergic receptors, such as propranolol and labetalol, are best suited to these circumstances. In an acute setting, these blockers can be administered intravenously. In a less critical situation, these drug can be given orally. A dose of 120 mg. to 240 mg. of propranolol per day in divided doses appears to work well to reduce spasms.

Calcium channel blockers also appear to have a beneficial effect on cocaine-induced vascular spasm. Nifedipine and verapamil are efficacious and can be given intravenously in the acute setting.[5]

When alcohol and cocaine are used together, a substance called "cocaethylene" is manufactured hepatically. Cocaethylene stimulates dopaminergic receptors. In a patient whose myocardium is vasoconstricted, dopaminergic stimulation can trigger a lethal event. The risk of sudden death is twenty-five times greater in persons who abuse cocaine and alcohol simultaneously, rather than cocaine alone.[6]

Although the effects on the cardiovascular system of both acute and chronic users of cocaine are well documented, the cessation of the drug does not appear to have any adverse effect on the cardiovascular system.

AMPHETAMINE & OTHER SYMPATHOMIMETICS

The sympathomimetics are a class of drugs that have long been commonly abused. Because of its ability to affect central nervous system stimulation after being ingested orally, amphetamine is the prototypical drug in this class which also includes methylene dioxymethamphetamine, methylphenidate, and khat.

Amphetamine, like cocaine, has the ability to raise both systolic and diastolic blood pressure. Although acting indirectly, amphetamine exerts this effect on blood pressure by altering catecholamine activity. Cardiac output, however, is not enhanced by amphetamine use. Although myocardial ischemia is unusual, amphetamine use does have multiple cardiovascular effects which appear to be dose related. These toxic effects include cephalgia, flushing, palpitation, cardiac arrhythmia, angina and hyper- or hypotension.

With the use of this class of drugs, cardiac rate is frequently increased. Relative hypoxia, due to increased cardiac rate, induces regional myocardial ischemia and subsequent cardiac arrhythmia.

Patients who present with a marked increase in cardiac rate, cardiac arrhythmias, or symptoms of coronary insufficiency must be monitored carefully. It is our recommendation that these patients be placed on a cardiac monitor and treated at least in an intermediate care setting.

Ventricular arrhythmias should be treated with appropriate intravenous therapy such as lidocaine. Amphetamine excretion can be enhanced by acidification of the urine. This will indirectly reduce cardiac symptoms. Since chlorpromazine directly antagonizes amphetamine activity, a trial dose of 25 to 50 mg. IV slow-push is recommended.

As with cocaine withdrawal, no cardiac sequelae, as a rule, occur. Long-term use can lead to high output failure and, on rare occasions, cardiomyopathy.

BENZODIAZEPINE

Benzodiazepine overdose causes only moderate depression of circulation. Large doses may cause a 15 to 20 percent decline in systolic blood pressure and vascular resistance. Changes in heart rate vary greatly from mild depression to tachycardia.

As benzodiazepines suppress respiration at higher dosages, generalized hypoxia may occur with subsequent induction of cardiac dysrhythmia. When patients present with a pulse oximetry of greater than 90 percent, cardiac telemetry and frequent intermittent determination of pulse oximetry is recommended. If the pulse oximeter is less than 90 percent, it is our recommendation that these patients be monitored in an intermediate or specialty-care area where continuous pulse oximetry and cardiac telemetry can be offered. If hypoxia and respiratory failure lead to the development of cardiac arrhythmia, ventilatory support will be needed.

Doxapram hydrochloride (Dopram) can be used to stimulate respiration. When given intravenously in low doses, it selectively stimulates respiration in normal human subjects, increasing both tidal volume and respiratory frequency.[7] Respiratory depression induced by benzodiazepine overdose rarely extends beyond 72 hours, at which time respiratory support can be withdrawn if the patient is stable.[8]

SEDATIVE-HYPNOTICS

Before the advent of more sophisticated recreational drugs, the sedative-hypnotics were widely abused both as single agents and in combination. In 1988, 6 percent of young adults reported nonmedical use of sedatives. Polydrug use further complicates the cardiac problems.

Sedatives and hypnotics used in therapeutically recommended doses have minimal effect on the cardiovascular system. When used in higher doses, the inhibitory effects on the cardiovascular system can produce profound hypotension. This hypotension is due to inhibition of ganglionic transmission, and to decreased cardiac output. This decrease causes increased peripheral resistance as well as increased cardiac rate.

The treatment for those patients is supportive. In milder cases, infusion of 0.9 N saline is sufficient. In more complicated cases, vascular support may require positive inotropic agents such as dobutamine HCl or dopamine HCl.

During withdrawal from these agents, generally no cardiac disturbances are observed. In patients who combine alcohol or amphetamines with sedative-hypnotics, we have observed ventricular ectopy during the early phases of patient withdrawal. These, as a rule, require no therapeutic intervention. However, these patients should be monitored on telemetry until stable.

ALCOHOL

Moderate amounts of ethanol consumption have relatively little effect on the cardiovascular system. Blood pressure, cardiac output and myocardial contraction do not significantly change. Cardiovascular depression observed in acute severe alcohol intoxication is due mainly to central vasomotor factors.[7]

Alcoholic cardiomyopathy is due to myocardial uptake of free fatty acids. Cardiomyopathy arising from alcohol abuse produces decreased cardiac output. The early symptoms closely resemble those of traditional congestive heart failure. This can be treated by sodium restriction, diuretics, and digitalization. As cardiac output continues to decline, cardiomyopathy becomes more refractory to digitalis therapy, making diuretics and angiotensin converting enzyme (ACE) inhibitors the mainstay of therapeutic intervention.

Withdrawal from ethanol in an acute setting is usually not associated with cardiovascular complications. However, after long-term use or excessive use of alcohol, both the direct and indirect effects on the cardiovascular system can be significant. These effects include congestive heart failure due to myocardial depression. Again, the use of sodium restriction, digitalis, diuretics and ACE inhibitors are indicated.

Chronic excessive use of alcohol can lead to malnutrition and many vitamin deficiencies. Hypomagnesemia is almost uniformly present. Hypomagnesemia can be corrected with an intravenous infusion of magnesium sulfate. Up to 40 grams can be infused per 24 hours. Usually a more modest dose of 4 to 6 grams intravenously every 8 hours will correct the most severe deficiency within 48 hours. For long-term chronic therapy, oral magnesium can be given.

Whether through dietary deficiency or metabolic dysfunction, hypokalemia is a well-known complication of chronic alcoholism. Replenishment can be accomplished by either oral or intravenous format. For oral therapy, a slow-release preparation such as K-Dur or Micro-K is employed. It is frequently necessary to correct the hypomagnesemia prior to adequate replenishing of the potassium deficiency, as adequate magnesium seems to play a role in potassium uptake.

All of these factors alone or in tandem can have disastrous effects on the cardiovascular system. These effects range from minimal performance abnormalities, to life-threatening dysrhythmia due to electrolyte imbalance, to fulminant congestive failure due to advanced cardiomyopathy. These electrolyte imbalances are of particular risk to those patients who have underlying coronary artery disease.

STEROIDS

In recent years, anabolic steroids have been abused to enhance physical performance and physique. The cardiovascular system is affected on a long-term basis primarily as a consequence of regulation of renal sodium excretion. These effects are seen in hypocorticism when reduction in blood volume, accompanied by increased viscosity, can lead to hypotension and cardiovascular collapse.[7]

These physiological changes are a result of the development of hyponatremia, hyperkalemia and cellular dehydration with contraction of the extracellular fluid volume. There is also an increase in capillary permeability and an inadequate vasomotor response of the small vessels to catecholamines. In addition to vascular changes, a reduction in cardiac size and output are noted.

Mineral corticoids promote sodium retention at the expense of potassium and hydrogen-ion excretion. This is due to stimulation of the renin-angiotensin system. The hypokalemia not only can effect cardiac performance, but can potentiate cardiac arrhythmias, particularly in a patient with coronary artery disease.

Hypertension arises from both the mineral corticoid and glucocorticoids. Mineral corticoids produce hypertension by renin-angiotensin stimulation. The hypertension that is glucocorticoid-induced is not well understood. The most plausible explanation is that cortisol-induced sodium retention promotes volume expansion and thus the hypertension.

With a steroid-induced cushingoid-like syndrome, withdrawal must be done slowly. The consequences of rapid withdrawal, particularly after long-term steroid abuse, can be life-threatening. Rapid withdrawal usually will result in hypocorticism which can lead to cardiovascular collapse.

Careful monitoring of serum cortisol should be a standard practice during withdrawal. Serum cortisol levels should be measured frequently during downward steroid titration. Patients should be observed for hypotensive pressure, orthostasis and general well-being. Since long-term suppression may result in the slow recovery of the pituitary axis, it would not be unusual for safe withdrawal from the drug to take six or more months.

CANNABOIDS

Marijuana exerts its major effects on the central nervous and cardiovascular systems. The most consistent cardiovascular effect is on blood pressure. Pressoreceptors maintain blood pressure by increasing the systolic blood pressure while supine, and decreasing blood pressure while standing. The rise in blood pressure is associated with an increased heart rate. Tachycardia of greater than 150 beats per minute is not uncommon. The increase in heart rate and supine systolic blood pressure is due, in part, to sympathetic stimulus by Δ-9-THC.

The increased heart rate results in increased oxygen demand. This demand can be especially hazardous in patients with coronary artery disease. The duration of exercise time tolerated before onset of angina is decreased substantially by smoking as little as one marijuana cigarette.[9]

Long-term smoking of marijuana can result in chronic bronchitis and perhaps asthma. These lung problems are induced by the tar produced by pyrolysis. Marijuana smoking is associated with the deposition of high amounts of particulate matter in the lungs. The deposition, over time, may lead to chronic respiratory disease, which can eventually lead to chronic hypoxia with development of cor pulmonale. In patients with coronary artery disease, chronic hypoxia aggravates ischemic heart disease and potentiates life-threatening dysrhythmia.

Heavy users of marijuana develop tolerance to its cardiac effects within a few days. Marijuana smoking or ingestion can produce a syndrome that includes multiple signs and symptoms but not major cardiovascular problems.[10] These withdrawal symptoms are short-lived and dissipate within four to five days (see Chapter 8, Marijuana).

NOTES

1. Abelson HI, Miller JD. A decade of trends in cocaine use in the household population. National Inst Drug Abuse Res Monogr Serv 1985; **61**:35-49.
2. Isner JM, Chokshi SK. Cocaine and vasopressant. NEJM 1989; **321**:1604-6.
3. Flores ED, Lang RA, Cigaprora RG, Hillis LD. Effect of cocaine on coronary artery disease; enhanced vasoconstriction at sites of significant stenosis. J Am College Cardiology 1990; **16**:74-9.
4. Bunn WH, Giannini AJ. Cardiovascular complications of cocaine abuse. Am Family Physician 1992; **46**:769-774.
5. Rangione AJ, Isner JM. Cocaine-induced contraction of vascular smooth muscle is inhibited by calcium channel blockade (abst.). J Am College Cardiology 1989; **13**:78A.
6. Grant BF, Hartford PC. Concurrent and simultaneous use of alcohol with cocaine: results of a national survey. Drug Alc Dependency 1990; **25**:97-104.
7. MacMahon SW, Blacket RB, MacDonald GJ. Obesity, alcohol consumption and blood pressure in Australian men and women. The National Heart Foundation of Australian risk factor prevalence study. J Hypertension 1984; **2**:85-91.
8. Calverley PM, Robson RH, Wraiphik TC, Prescottle RM, Flenley DC. The ventilatory effects of doxapram in normal man. Clin Sci 1983; **65**:65-69.
9. Hollister LE. Health aspects of cannabis. Pharmacol Rev 1986; **38**:1-20.
10. Jones RT, Benowitzen JG, Bachman J. Clinical studies of cannabis tolerance and dependency. Ana NY Acad Sci 1976; **282**:221-239.

CHAPTER 17

DUAL DIAGNOSIS PATIENTS

The definition of the dual diagnosis patient varies from author to author. Dual diagnosis can be considered to be the presence of two coexisting diseases, one of psychiatric genesis and one of chemical dependency. Alternately, chemical dependency can be thought to be a function of a primary psychiatric illness. In this school of thought, patients are seen to be abusing drugs to self-medicate their core psychiatric illness such as depression or anxiety. A third school of thought holds that the psychiatric disorder and the drug abuse are genetically, and therefore biochemically, linked. Finally, the chemical dependency disorder may be viewed to the primary illness and the disorder of mood, thought or personality as a direct result of the addictive process through either biochemical (e.g., alteration of neurotransmitters, neuropathies, nutritional disorders) or sociological (e.g., drug-seeking behavior, acts performed while intoxicated) vectors.

Regardless of which school of thought is most applicable, the impact of each disorder upon the other increases the severity of expression of both disorders. This increase in severity is so great that it becomes a difference in kind. Since this book is a review of current thought in the diagnosis and treatment of drugs of abuse, the content will be inclusive rather than exclusive. All four schools of thought will be incorporated into the following discussion.[1]

Because of the complex interrelationship between chemical dependency and psychiatric disorders, it is impossible to practice either psychiatry or addiction-ology in isolation. At one time in their lives, 74 percent of all psychiatric patients have abused drugs. Of these, 13 percent go on to be drug addicts while another 15-20 percent become alcoholics.[2] Twenty-five percent of all men presenting with impotence have a drug or alcoholic disorder. Nearly half of all inpatient substance abuse patients have a depressive disorder while another 5 to 10 percent have a schizophrenic or schizophreniform disorder.[3]

The relapse rate for psychiatric patients with an untreated major chemical dependency disorder is nearly three-times that of psychiatric patients with a treated chemical disorder. For substance-abusing populations, the rate of relapse for untreated co-existing psychiatric illness is approximately five-times that of the treated population.[4]

In applying the label of dual diagnosis, it is necessary to first detoxify the patient and allow sufficient time for the symptoms of intoxication, addiction and detoxification to remit. In the case of alcoholics presenting with a dual diagnosis of dysphoria, 70 percent of male or female patients are cured of their depressive disease three to four weeks after detoxification.[5] This cure occurs in the absence of any biochemical psychotherapeutic intervention. While it is generally accepted that a finite time period must elapse, there is great controversy as to the extent of this period. Generally, most researchers agree that it is three to four weeks, however, acceptance of this time interval is not universal.

Complicating the development of a specific time-protocol are the nutritional, traumatic and other deficiencies caused by the addiction.[3] In designing a pharmacological treatment modality, the clinician must have intimate knowledge of the biochemical pathology causing the psychiatric disorder as well as the biochemical pathology resulting from the drug abuse. In many cases, these pathologies may be genetically linked to such disorders as alcoholism, sympathomimetic abuse (in depression) and anticholinergic abuse (in schizophrenia). Certainly in using this knowledge, drugs that relieve the psychiatric illness, as well as reduce the cravings and the psychiatric symptoms, can be intelligently applied.

Ideally, the medication prescribed should treat both the psychiatric illness and the effects of the drugs of abuse. These effects can either be the addiction itself, the withdrawal symptoms, or the psychiatric sequelae. These sequelae may be the depression seen in chronic psychedelic and sympathomimetic abuse, or the anxiety associated with alcoholic patients.

AFFECTIVE DISORDERS

The most commonly studied interrelationship of dual diagnosis is that between alcoholism and major depression. There is a 75 percent prevalence of depression in alcoholic men and women. Men with bipolar disorder have a similar prevalence of approximately 50 percent.[6]

There seems to be genetic linkage indicating a relationship between major depression and alcoholism. Families of patients with a dual diagnosis of alcoholism and depression have a similar rate of risk for depression as do families of patients with alcoholism only.[7] The reverse of this relationship, however, is not true. Dual diagnosis patients have families with an increased risk of alcoholism in comparison to families of patients who have a diagnosis of depression only. As a result, it can be concluded that alcoholism is a possible factor in triggering general depression.

Although depression is the primary factor in patients with a dual diagnosis of alcoholism/depression, the depression can be related in expression to sequelae of depression. Alcoholism can cause depletion of financial resources, alienation of family members, personality disintegration secondary to central neuropathy, and disruption of the patient's social matrix. Also, the direct effects of alcohol such as hypomagnesemia, niacin deficiency, Wernicke-Korsakoff syndrome, vitamin B-12 and folic acid deficiency, and albumin deficiency can all produce dysphoric symptomatology. The primary depressives, however, have an earlier age of onset of depression than alcoholics in whom the depression is a secondary rather than primary cause.[8]

Treatment of depressed alcoholics is based upon current knowledge of the multiple receptor-site activity of alcohol, as well as the serotonergic and noradrenergic bases of depression and mania. Several studies have demonstrated that 50 percent of dual diagnosis alcohol/depressive patients report decreased craving for alcohol with imipramine.[9] Similar findings have been reported for most of the serotonergic reuptake inhibitors in smaller open studies.

Opioid-addicted depressive patients respond with decreased dysphoria, decreased anxiety, and decreased craving for opiates when treated with doxepin.[10] The depression associated with opioid addiction, however, seems to be a secondary rather than a primary result or independent factor.

In contrast, the depression associated with cocaine addiction can either be primary to the cocaine addiction, a result of the addiction, or an aggravation of the underlying depression.[10] Desipramine and maprotiline have been reported to be useful in reducing cocaine cravings and post withdrawal addiction.[11]

Little is known of the interrelationship between affective disorders and the psychedelic agents but the serotonergic reuptake inhibitors fluoxetine and paroxetine are useful in treating depression in these groups.

The mania of bipolars who abuse alcohol may be treated with large amounts of magnesium sulfate. Many alcoholics manifest hypomagnesemia due to nutritional inattention. Hypomagnesemia can create a pseudo-manic state or precipitate manic symptoms in bipolar patients. Although some researchers at the beginning of the twentieth century reported a reduction of manic symptoms and a reduction of alcoholic craving with magnesium, later research has not borne the accuracy of these findings.

Anxiety Disorders

Anxiety disorders are difficult to treat in dual diagnosis patients since chronic prescription of potentially addicting benzodiazepines must, of necessity, be avoided. Although many protocols advise the use of serotonergic reuptake inhibitors, this subjects the patient to a long latency period. In many drug treatment programs, the patient is kept drug-free for 3 to 4 weeks after detoxification, enduring anxiety and panic symptoms before the medication is prescribed. After initiation of treatment, the SRI's usually require 2 to 4 weeks before the patient notes anxiolytic onset. By this time, many patients simply give up. To reduce this unwanted relapse, benztropine, or beta-blockers such as atenolol or propranolol, can be prescribed until the SRI-anxiolysis is produced. In patients with combined depression, anxiety and substance abuse disorder, the short time interval of beta-blocker intake is usually insufficient to aggravate the depression.

Personality Disorders

By an elastic definition, all chemically dependent patients can be thought to have a personality disorder, either an addictive personality or frank sociopathy. Using the definitions of DSM-III-R, DSM-IV or ICD-9-CM, 20 percent of all male and 5 to 10 percent of all female addicts including alcoholics are seen to be "antisocial." These patients are difficult to treat in an inpatient psychiatric unit. Research into nonverbal communication and small group dynamics shows these dual diagnosis sociopathic/chemically dependent patients to be particularly adept in polarizing and disrupting inpatient psychiatric milieux.[12]

Schizophrenia

Nearly 40 percent of all schizophrenic patients treated with required inpatient hospitalization have a history of substance abuse.[13]

Anticholinergic abuse is found almost exclusively under this psychiatric diagnosis.[3] The patient generally discovers anticholinergics when they are prescribed concomitantly with phenothiazine or butyrophenone neuroleptics to reduce symptoms of secondary Parkinsonism. Because of relief of many negative symptoms of schizophrenia, patients generally continue to use anticholinergics in prescribed or excess amounts. This use is continued even after the neuroleptic is discontinued either by the physician or by the patient.

In addition to anticholinergic drugs, there is a possible linkage between alcoholism and schizophrenia. The serotonergic activity which may be responsible for the negative symptoms of schizophrenia may also be linked to alcoholic cravings. The serontonergic-dopaminergic neuroleptics, clozapine and risperidone, both share serotonergic activity and have been reported to be effective in reducing alcoholic cravings in dual diagnosis schizophrenic/alcoholic patients. Naltrexone, which is indicated for the reduction of alcoholic cravings, has been reported to reduce the "positive" symptoms of schizophrenia in these dual-diagnosis patients.[14]

The negative symptoms of schizophrenia are self-treated by some schizophrenics with cocaine and the sympathomimetics. The antidepressants maprotiline and desipramine, used to reduce post-withdrawal cravings, can also reduce the negative symptoms of schizophrenia. Schizophrenic patients who experience exacerbation of their psychosis with phencyclidine are best treated with risperidone which, in addition to its DA-2 dopaminergic activity, also acts at serotonergic receptor sites.[15] Although not yet reported, respiridone may prove equally effective in treating schizophrenics who acutely or chronically abuse psychedelic agents.

Obsessive Compulsive Disorders (OCD)

Chemical dependency may one day be proven to be a variant of obsessive compulsive disorder (OCD). OCD is often self-treated with alcohol. Clomipramine and fluvoxamine are commonly prescribed to treat obsessive behavior but, unfortunately, no double-blind studies have been published supporting these agents in treating any chemical dependency.

Eating Disorders

It has been reported that 20 percent of all bulimics are alcoholic or otherwise drug dependent. Possibly another 5 percent of all anorectics are also drug dependent, predominantly upon sympathomimetics because of there anorectic effects. Serotonergic reuptake inhibitors have been useful for depressive bulimics but, unfortunately, there is no pharmacological agent which has similar efficacy for anorexia.

Attention Deficit Hyperactivity Disorder

The literature is sparse on diagnosis and treatment of co-existing attention deficit hyperactivity disorder (ADHD) and substance abuse disorder. However, 30 percent of all children continue to manifest ADHD into adulthood. It is in this adult population that 25 percent of drug abuse occurs. Within this group, 15 to 45 percent abuse alcohol and between 10 to 50 percent abuse or are addicted to other psychoactive drugs.[16]

Because of the underlying diagnosis, psychoactive drugs such as methylphenidate, pemoline and amphetamines are prescribed with extreme caution, if at all.[17] These patients are at very high risk for sympathomimetic abuse. Clonidine, an alpha-adrenergic agonist, can reduce symptoms of ADHD as well as modulate opiate, alcohol and sympathomimetic withdrawal and cravings. The beta-blockers, verapamil, and the tricyclic antidepressants, can all serve a similar function.[18] Preliminary work indicates that venlafaxine, which acts at serotonergic and noradrenergic receptors, can also be effective.[19]

CONCLUSION

There has been and continues to be an unfortunate polarization of the treatment of dual diagnosis patients, even when both diagnoses have been accurately made. The patient tends to be pulled between two groups. One type of mental health group treats the psychiatric disorder primarily and concentrates secondarily on the psychopathological etiology of the addiction without actually treating the addiction itself. Antithetically, there are chemical dependency groups which promote abstinence and either ignore the coexisting psychiatric illness or actively discourage psychotherapeutic or psychopharmacologic treatment. Recently, psychiatry has attempted to bridge the therapeutic chasm between these two groups by integrating psychopathology with chemical dependency.

Psychiatrists who treat drug addicts, or psychiatric patients with drug illnesses, should coordinate treatment with drug rehabilitation programs. They must not fall into the trap of viewing psychotherapy as a treatment of the drug addiction, or of seeing the peer-support system of chemical dependency programs as a substitute for psychotherapy.

It should go without saying that scheduled drugs should never be prescribed for these groups. However, this should not obviate rigorous treatment with nonaddicting psychotropic medication.

Treatment of the dual diagnosis patient is difficult because of the complexity of treating two concurrent illnesses. This difficulty is further aggravated by competing treatment philosophies: the conflicts between the nonmedical professionals subscribing to either philosophy; and the patient's reaction to the active opposition between the two groups of treating professionals. This opposition can be aggravated further by the manipulative strategies substance abusers often employ. It is therefore incumbent upon the clinician to attend to both diseases, the patient, and the sometimes competing philosophies of the various members of the treatment team.

NOTES

1. Giannini AJ. Drug abuse and depression: catecholamine depletion suggested as biological tie between cocaine withdrawal and depression. Natl Inst Drug Abuse Notes 1987; **2(2)**:5.
2. Schuckit MA. Genetic and clinical implications of alcoholism and affective disorders. Am J Psychiatry 1986; **143**:140-147.
3. Giannini AJ, Collins GB, Substance abuse and thought disorders. In: Gold MA, Slaby AE (Eds.), Dual Diagnosis Patients. New York: Marcel-Dekker, 1991.
4. Agency for Health Care Policy Research. Depression in Primary Care. Rockville: Nat Inst Health, 1993.
5. Mirin SM, Weiss RD, Michael J. Affective illness in substance abusers: Community Epidemiology Work Group Proceedings - II. NIDA Rockville, 1984.

6. Weissman MM, Meyers JK. Clinical depression in alcoholism. Am J Psychiatry 1980; **137**:372-373.
7. Schuekit MA. Alcoholic patients with secondary diagnosis. Am J Psychiatry 1983; **140**:711-714.
8. Jekel JF, Allen DF. Trends in drug abuse. Yale J Biol Med 1987; **60**:45-52.
9. Lumeng L, Wong DT, Threlkeld M. Neuronal receptors for alcohol and nonalcohol preferring rats. Third Cong Int Soc Biomed Res Alcohol (abst). Helsinki, June 1986.
10. Giannini AJ, Malone DA, Giannini MC, Price WA, Loiselle RH. Treatment of chronic cocaine and phencyclidine abuse with desipramine. J Clin Pharmacology 1986; **26**:211-215.
11. Gawin FM, Kleber HD. Cocaine abuse treatment: open pilot trial with desipramine and lithium carbonate. Arch Gen Psychiatry 1984; **41**:903-904.
12. Giannini AJ, DeFrance DT, Loiselle RH, Giannini MC. Reception of nonverbal communication in alcoholics. J Gen Psychol 1984; **116**:241-244.
13. NIMH Epidemiological Cachement Area Household Survey. 1980-1985, Rockville: NIMH, 1985.
14. Volpicelli JR, Clay KL, Watson NJ, O'Brien CP: Naltrexone in the treatment of alcoholism. J Clin Psychiatry 1995; **56(S7)**:39-44.
15. Gabbert JF, Giannini AJ. Risperidone treatment of acute phencyclidine intoxication. Am J Therapeutics. (In press.)
16. Weiss G. Attention Deficit Hyperactivity Disorder. Philadelphia: WB Sanders, 1992.
17. Khantzian EJ, Gawin FH, Fiordan C, Kleber HD. Methylphenidate treatment of cocaine dependence. J Subst Abuse Treatment 1984; **1**:107-112.
18. Price WA, Giannini AJ, Krishen A. Management of acute PCP intoxication with verapamil Clin Toxicol 1986; **24**:85-86.
19. Wilens TE, Biederman J, Spencer TJ. Venlafaxine for adult ADHD (ltr). Am J Psychiatry 1995; **152**:1099-1100.

CHAPTER 18

TREATING PREGNANT AND NURSING DRUG ABUSERS

All drugs of abuse are able to exert their effects because they are capable of crossing the blood-brain barrier by the mechanism of passive diffusion. In passive diffusion, the drug moves down the gradient until equilibrium is maintained between the central nervous system and the periphery. This diffusion can be modified by numerous factors including differential protein binding and metabolism. Unfortunately, the blood-brain barrier, which allows centrally active drugs to pass through it, is similar in construction to the placental membranes. Therefore, any drug which can pass into the brain can also pass through the placenta into the developing child. Also, all centrally active drugs can pass into the lactating ducts and into the mother's milk.

Because of the facility by which drugs can reach the developing or nursing child, a special problem presents itself to the treatment team when a pregnant or nursing addict is under its care. This problem is not an isolated one. Nearly 60 percent of all pregnant women use alcohol at some time during the pregnancy, and up to 3 to 10 percent meet the diagnostic criteria for alcoholism.[1] Ten to thirty percent of all pregnant women use marijuana and 5 to 15 percent use some form of cocaine or other stimulant.[2] Treatment teams isolated from addiction such as the general maternity unit can expect that nearly 25 percent of their patients will have used drugs or excess alcohol at some time during the pregnancy.[3]

This is further compounded by the tendency of addicts to not seek prenatal care. Only 12 percent of pregnant addicts involve themselves in any sort of early prenatal care, although another 10 to 12 percent do receive some cursory care, usually in the third trimester.[4]

As a result of chemical abuse and maternal neglect of the developing baby, the neonate is at multiple risk. Primary risks include direct teratogenic effects of the drug and postpartum withdrawal symptoms.[5] In addition, there are secondary effects including spontaneous abortion due to uterine contractility or abruptio placentae, breech birth, and eclampsia.

There is also a risk of AIDS and hepatitis through the use of contaminated needles or the increased promiscuity of this population. The baby is particularly vulnerable to all these illnesses because of: the plasticity of the embryonic and fetal tissue; the inability of the fetus to metabolize most drugs of abuse until the third trimester; hypoalbuminemia with diminished protein binding in the maternal circulatory system; and the diminished maternal renal clearance that occurs with pregnancy. In addition to these general effects, there are many specific effects for each of the drugs of abuse.

ALCOHOL

The major teratogenic effects of alcohol occur in women who generally abuse 5 ounces of 200 proof alcohol-equivalents daily, on a regular or semi-regular basis during the first trimester (for example, 10 shots of whiskey, 10 glasses of wine, or a six-pack of beer per day). The baby with fetal alcohol syndrome presents with microcephaly, shortened palpebral fissures, diminished birth weight, diminished length, and facial dysmorphosis. Other common birth defects occur in the cardiac septum, the skeleton, the urogenital system (especially in males), and in the central nervous system.

While fetal alcohol syndrome does not occur in alcoholics who abstained during the pregnancy, the babies' average birth weight is approximately 250 grams less than in babies born to nonalcoholic mothers. This compares with alcoholic mothers who do not abstain and give birth to children who are, on the average, 500 grams smaller. This impaired growth tends to continue throughout life. Children of alcoholic mothers tend to be shorter than those of nonalcoholic mothers.

In addition to teratogenic effects, there is a neonatal withdrawal syndrome which usually manifests itself at 6 to 12 hours postpartum. It includes irritability which may progress to seizures. There is diminished suck reflex, hypotonicity, and hypersensitivity to sound and light. Generally, this withdrawal is considered a medical emergency and is treated with benzodiazepines.

BENZODIAZEPINES

Benzodiazepines exert their teratogenic effect on the central nervous system. The child may present with hypertonicity or frank floppy infant syndrome. The symptoms of benzodiazepine withdrawal in infants are similar to that of an adult. There are tremors, hypotonicity or hypertonicity, and the possibility of frank seizures. Detoxification is accomplished by benzodiazepines or barbiturate in liquid drop form.[6]

COCAINE

The major risk for cocaine abusers is spontaneous abortion through abruptio placentae. Cocaine is a sympathomimetic. Its actions on the biogenic amines cause increased intensity and frequency of uterine contractions, which diminish blood flow to the placenta and the infant. Mothers who chronically use cocaine subject their children to the fetal cocaine syndrome. These children are known as crack babies. They tend to be small and hyper-irritable with diminished coordination and a diminished Moro response. As life progresses, they tend to be of below-average intelligence, hyperkinetic, and late in achieving normal growth milestones.[7]

PHENCYCLIDINE

The dissociatives work upon the central nervous system. Babies born to phencyclidine-addicted mothers tend to be labile and nonresponsive to the environment. They have generalized tremor, diminished strength, hyperreflexia, and diminished Moro reflex. At times, they also manifest hyperbilirubinemia.[8]

MARIJUANA

The major psychoactive ingredient of marijuana, Δ-9-tetrahydrocannabinol (THC), accumulates in the fetal central nervous system. The major effects are dose related, so that the more the mother indulges, the greater the limitations of birth weight, birth length and head size. Babies of mothers who consistently use marijuana tend to be hyper-irritable, tremulous and nonreactive to visual stimuli. Because of the effects of marijuana, there is a risk for spontaneous abortion and premature birth.[9]

OPIATES

Opiates act on ectodermic, endodermic and mesodermic tissue. They also cause fetal opiate syndrome which presents with cyanosis, intracranial hemorrhage, hyaline membrane disease, hypobilirubinemia, hypocalcemia, hypomagnesemia and septicemia.

Neonatal withdrawal syndrome occurs within 12 to 36 hours postpartum. In addition to the usual withdrawal effects found in the adult addicts, the neonate manifest increased finger sucking, diminished Moro reflex and sneezing. Within the neonatal withdrawal syndrome, there is a respiratory tetrad including apnea, intermittent cyanosis, intercostal muscle retraction and tachypnea.

Opiate-addicted babies are generally detoxified with paregoric or chlorpromazine. The use of benzodiazepines and barbiturates for detoxification has been reported in the literature but, unfortunately, these medications can be associated with respiratory depression.[10]

PSYCHEDELICS

There is no well-documented study of teratogenic or withdrawal effects of maternal psychedelic abuse. There are, however, case reports of abnormalities of the lens, retina and cornea; of cardiac and spinal defects; and of spontaneous abortion.[11]

SEDATIVES

Sedative abuse is associated again with low birth weight and height, prematurity, and facial dysmorphosis. This dysmorphosis is sometimes confused with fetal alcohol syndrome. Withdrawal symptoms occur 6 to 12 days postpartum and are treated with benzodiazepines on a slow-withdrawal basis.[12]

SYMPATHOMIMETICS

The teratogenic effects of sympathomimetics include palatine and cardiac cushion defects. The infant is most likely to develop these defects if drug abuse occurs during the first trimester. The sympathomimetic withdrawal syndrome is similar to that of cocaine.[13]

NURSING MOTHER

In many cases, the mother remains addicted throughout the pregnancy because of the tendency for addicts not to seek prenatal care. As a result, the emergency room staff or the maternity staff is left to deliver the addicted mother without history or preparation, on an emergency basis. After the birth, she becomes a "captive patient" and is usually detoxified.

In cases where the drug-abusing mother does come in for prenatal care, however, detoxification may be withheld. This is because of the danger of greater damage to the fetus, or of spontaneous abortion during the withdrawal process. In either circumstance, the staff is left to detoxify the new mother as well as the child.

In many cases there is an attempt to promote bonding by encouraging the mother to nurse the infant. This may be done in accordance with the wishes of the mother, or in compliance with hospital philosophy. However, if the mother is experiencing withdrawal from any type of psychoactive drug, this is to be avoided at all cost. Any substance given to the mother during the detoxification period will inevitably pass into the mammary glands. Here it will be concentrated at levels much higher than that in the maternal blood. This concentration occurs because of mammary gland action and the disparity between maternal and infant size.[14]

If it is in the child's best interest to promote bonding, the mother should be encouraged to hold and feed her child. If the mother is going through a withdrawal process, staff members should be available to assist her if withdrawal symptoms, especially those of tremors and hyper-irritability, manifest themselves.

If the mother keeps the child, one of the goals of psychotherapy is to transmute the addict/drug bond into a maternal/child bond. Although this is obvious, it is often neglected. Children of addicts are subject to a high degree of parental neglect and parental abuse. They tend to have a higher rate of addiction, suicide attempts, and failure to thrive than children of nonaddicting parents. In addition, these children are more challenging because of the numerous teratogenic drug syndromes. The drug-abusing mother, who is ill-equipped to take care of her own emotional needs, finds it difficult to raise an emotionally, intellectually or physically challenged child.[15]

NOTES

1. Sukal RJ, Miller NS, Reel G. Alcohol abuse during pregnancy. Alcoholism 1990; **4**:134-140.
2. Chasnoff IJ, Landress H, Barrett M. The Pinellas County study. Annual Meeting Natl Assoc Perinatal Addict Res Educ. Miami: September 20, 1989.
3. U.S. Dept HHS. Res Monograph. Women and Alcohol. Washington, DC: DHHS Publ No (ADM) 80-835, 1986.
4. US Dept HHS Res Monograph. Women and Alcohol DHHS (ADM) 86-1139, Washington DC, 1988.
5. Keshavan MS, Kennedy JS. Drug-Induced Dysfunction in Psychiatry. New York: Hemisphere, 1992.
6. Winship KA, Cabal DA, Weber JCP, Griffen JP. Maternal drug histories and central nervous system anomalies. Arch Dis Childhood 1984; **59**:1052-1060.
7. Chasnoff IJ, Burns WJ, Schroull SH, Giannini MRC. Cocaine use in pregnancy NEJM 1985; **313**:666-667.
8. Giannini AJ. PCP: detecting the abusers. Med Aspects Human Sexuality 1987; **21(1)**:100-108.
9. Bloodworth RC. Medical problems associated with marijuana abuse. Psychiatric Med 1987; **3**:173-184.
10. Chasnoff IJ. Newborn infants with drug withdrawal symptoms. Pediatr Rev 1990; **9**:273-277.
11. Rovini IM, Nistri CN, Bausi L. Tossicomania e pediatrica. Ricercea è Salute. 1994; **29(6)**:14-21.
12. Chasnoff IJ. Drug use in pregnancy. Ped Clin North Am 1988; **35**:1403-12.
13. Dixon S. Effects of transplacental exposure to cocaine and methamphetamine on the neonate. West J Med 1989; **150**:436-442.
14. Kaufman KR, Petrosky RA, Pitts FN. PCP in amniotic fluid and breast milk. J Clin Psychiatry 1983; **44**:296-297.
15. Deren S. Children of substance abusers. J Subst Abuse Treatment 1987; **3**:77-94.

CHAPTER 19

NUTRITIONAL ASPECTS OF DRUG ABUSE

Almost anyone addicted to drugs or alcohol is malnourished in one form or another, whether underweight or overweight. Once an addict decides to seek help and end the addiction, the process of healing can begin. As in any healing process, proper nutrition is a basic component of care. All drug and alcohol abusers can be considered at high nutritional risk.

ALCOHOL

Alcohol abuse creates altered ingestion, digestion, absorption, metabolism and excretion patterns. Alcoholics are usually low or deficient in vitamin A (retinol), vitamin B1 (thiamine), vitamin B2 (riboflavin), vitamin B6 (pyridoxine), vitamin B12 (cyanocobalamine), vitamin C (ascorbic acid), vitamin D (calciferol), vitamin E (tocopherol), folate, magnesium and zinc. These deficiencies occur due to a direct effect on the liver cells which activate these vitamins.

Food will stay in the stomach for a while, waiting to be digested, but alcohol refuses to wait. Alcohol is not digested, but rather is absorbed directly throughout the gastrointestinal tract.

Although alcohol affects every organ in the body, its primary target is the liver. The liver normally has a very organized systematic routine of taking in excess fatty acids and shipping these out into the body as triglycerides. Liver cells preferentially metabolize alcohol. However, in cases of excessive alcohol intake, the fatty acids are left waiting, relentlessly accumulating and destroying liver cells in the process.

Alcohol dehydrogenase is a hepatic enzyme which oxidizes alcohol. If the concentration of alcohol overwhelms the amount of available alcohol dehydrogenase, the excess alcohol will enter into circulation. It will then recirculate until liver enzymes are available to convert it to acetaldehyde.

The amount of available enzymes is partially dependent upon the amount of food in the alimentary tract. In like manner, the rate of alcohol absorption is inversely proportional to the amount of food in the stomach. Also, high amounts of carbohydrates or fats further reduce the rate of absorption. One of the first tolls alcohol abuse exacts from the liver is a condition known as fatty liver. A decrease in the supply of available protein reduces the production of lipoprotein. This, in turn, reduces oxygen and nutrient distribution to the cells.[1]

In alcohol abusers, the small intestine purges or destroys the nutrients within it. Thiamine, zinc and magnesium are most easily lost. A deficiency in thiamine produces Wernicke's encephalopathy. This is a syndrome characterized by amnestic episodes (blackouts), leg cramps, mydriasis, blepharospasm, nystagmus and amblyopia. Thiamine is needed for growth, carbohydrate metabolism, and the proper functioning of nerves and muscles. A diet that regularly includes brewer's yeast, wheat germ, whole grain products, nuts, sunflower seeds and liver will increase thiamine levels. As the typical alcoholic does not usually consume these foods on a regular basis, therapeutic dosages may be prescribed in the beginning of recovery. The usual dosages are 100 to 200 mg. every day, intramuscularly. This dosage is followed by thiamine 200 mg. every day, orally, for 2 to 6 months.

Magnesium depletion occurs through urinary excretion during periods of alcohol ingestion. This particular depletion may be the cause of the irritability experienced after a prolonged bout of drinking. Other symptoms of deficiency include anxiety, fasciculations, formications and hallucinations, usually of small bugs. The recommended daily allowance of magnesium oxide for women is 280 mg, and is 350 mg. for men. This may initially be prescribed in supplemental form—by pill or injection. However, it is easily administered through the diet. A high-magnesium diet should include generous portions of soybeans, brown rice, legumes, green leafy vegetables, nuts, peanuts, whole grains and chocolate. Acute treatment of severe hypomagnesemia is in the form of magnesium sulfate intravenously or intramuscularly.

Zinc is necessary for the growth and repair of the liver, and maintenance of olfactory and gustatory sensations. This mineral is responsible for the regeneration of the damaged liver after discontinuance of excess alcohol intake. The poor dietary habits associated with alcoholism can lead to a zinc deficiency. Meat, liver, oysters, fish, wheat germ, and nuts are all excellent sources of zinc. Treatment dosage is zinc oxide, 15 mg. every day.[2]

Most alcoholics have a general deficiency of many or all members of the "B" vitamin group. Vitamin B12 is required for the metabolism of high quantities of alcohol and for the repair of damaged tissues. Severe deficiencies of B12 can result in peripheral nerve damage, also known as the syndrome of alcoholic polyneuropathy. Symptoms include numbness and diminished vibratory sense. Macrocytic anemia can also occur. A diet rich in animal foods such as liver, chicken, fish and beef will help to increase amounts of vitamin B12. A related vitamin, folic acid, is used for cell replication. Deficiency of folic acid leads to impairment of DNA and protein synthesis. Foods such as broccoli, spinach, asparagus, and liver contain sufficient amounts of folic acid.[2]

Initial treatment usually includes vitamin B12 1 to 2 cc intramuscularly, followed by 1 mg. of folic acid per day. Interestingly, beer drinkers have a reduced rate of polyneuropathy due to the high amount of folate naturally found in this beverage.

Vitamin B2 (riboflavin) can be found in such dairy products as milk, cheese and yogurt. Almonds, brewer's yeast, broccoli, liver, wheat germ and wild rice also contain riboflavin. Deficiency of this vitamin can cause depression, psychotic behavior, lethargy and anhedonia.[3] As little as 10 mg. every day, orally, can reduce all symptoms.

Vitamin B6 assists in red blood cell formation, maintenance of brain function, and protein utilization. Higher protein intake requires increased vitamin B6. A deficiency in B6 causes abnormal central nervous system function, including neuritis, hyper-irritability, and convulsions. Vitamin B6 can be found in brewer's yeast, brown rice, sunflower seeds, bananas, broccoli, liver and salmon.

Vitamin C is the sunshine vitamin. It is popularly used to treat a wide variety of problems such as stress-related ailments, hypertension, diarrhea, hypoxia, insomnia, shingles, upper respiratory infections, mental illness, headache, constipation, arthritis, bursitis, gout, cramps, allergies, bronchitis, halitosis, gastritis and free-radical formation. Vitamin C-rich foods include broccoli, green peppers, cabbage, melons and citrus fruits. Alcoholics require high doses of vitamin C, usually 2 to 3 times the Recommended Daily Allowance of 60 mg. every day.[4]

Alcohol abusers often suffer from diarrhea. This creates a loss of water, electrolytes and fat-soluble vitamins. The fat-soluble vitamins include vitamins A, D, E, and K.

Vitamin A can be found in liver, carrots, broccoli, apricots, sweet potatoes and spinach. The main function of vitamin A is to promote good vision by generating pigments necessary for retina functioning. This is especially helpful for seeing in dim light. Vitamin A also helps form and maintain healthy skin, teeth, mucous membranes and skeletal and soft tissues by antioxidant action. Vitamin A may also be essential for lactation in pregnant women and for reproduction. If replacement is indicated, prescribe beta-carotene, 5,000 UV. every day.[1]

Vitamin D is easily obtained in milk, fortified grain products, oysters, fish, cheese, margarine and from exposure to the sun—sunshine converts cholesterol to vitamin D. Vitamin D promotes the absorption of calcium, helping to maintain proper blood levels of calcium and phosphorus. A deficiency of this vitamin can lead to rickets.

Vitamin E sources include vegetable oils (soybean, cottonseed, sunflower, corn) and margarine. In addition, wheat germ, corn, nuts, seeds, olives, asparagus, spinach and other green leafy vegetables contain large amounts of vitamin E. Treatment with 75 I.U. of vitamin E each day is usually sufficient, and will aid in the utilization of vitamin K, which promotes clotting. Colonic bacteria provide about 80 percent of the necessary vitamin K we need; the rest must come from our diet. Sources of vitamin K include cabbage, cauliflower, spinach and other leafy vegetables, cereals and oils, particularly soybean oil. Daily replacement dosage of vitamin K is 30 mg. orally.

An alcoholic's calcium and potassium levels may also be low or at near depletion levels, depending upon the extent of alcohol abuse and dietary habits.[5] Calcium is needed to activate cAMP, (cyclic amino monophosphate). It is also necessary for neuronal transmission, muscular contraction, blood clotting, and as a building element of bones and teeth. Sources of calcium include milk and milk products, green leafy vegetables, citrus fruits, dried peas, beans, sardines and shellfish.

Potassium is found in bananas, dried fruits, peanut butter, potatoes and orange juice. Potassium, along with sodium, helps regulate body fluid balance, and aids in the transmission of nerve impulses. Heavy drinkers may be low in potassium due to poor diet or alcohol-induced diarrhea. Inadequate amounts of potassium can produce muscular weakness. Oral replacement of potassium is advised.

In the general treatment of alcoholism, high-protein diets and large amounts of the B vitamins should be prescribed. High protein foods include meat, chicken, liver, fish, eggs, cheese, vegetables, milk and grains. It is very important to maintain regularly scheduled meals, for sudden lowering of blood levels sugar can trigger a craving for alcohol.[6]

BARBITURATES

When withdrawal from barbiturates is initiated, the patient is weak, anxious, nauseous, and/or tremulous. For two to five days the patient may be quite sick, with recurrences of delirium tremens and gastric distress. The patient is usually weaned with a short-acting barbiturate or long-acting phenobarbital to avoid grand mal-type seizures from withdrawal.

Since chronic use of barbiturates also raises the body's need for vitamin C, this vitamin should be a part of the detoxification process. In addition to relying on dietary sources, we have found 300 mg. of vitamin C daily, administered orally, is useful in reducing the severity of symptoms.[7]

MARIJUANA

Marijuana is associated with an increased appetite usually within several minutes of the initial high. During such episodes, commonly known as the munchies, marijuana smokers usually eat junk foods of low nutrient density, mainly sweets. Very heavy use of marijuana has been associated with temporary intestinal disorders such as diarrhea, abdominal cramping and inflammation. However, it does not seem to have any long-term effect on the gastrointestinal tract.

To nutritionally treat a marijuana abusers, one would have to review the symptoms. For cramping and diarrhea, a low fat, low fiber diet would be suggested. The recovering addict should be advised to eat baked, broiled, or roasted foods, yogurt, mild cheeses, cooked or canned fruits, fruit and vegetable juices, refined enriched bread, cooked cereals, noodles, and crackers. A number of other foods should be prohibited, including fried foods, whole fruits and berries, raw vegetables, legumes, whole grain products, aged cheeses, coconut, nuts, bran and seeds.

AMPHETAMINES AND DIET PILLS

Amphetamines and over-the-counter diet pills produce a hyper-alertness and a decrease in appetite. Many brands of diet pills are available on grocery store shelves, while others are physician-prescribed amphetamines. The use of diet pills to lose weight is an unhealthy methodology. Generally, any weight lost in this manner is temporary and regained when normal eating resumes.

During detoxification, the metabolic rate may fall. To avoid this eventuality, large doses of vitamin C and high complex-carbohydrate diet is advised. With this diet, sodium intake should be monitored.[8]

COCAINE

Cocaine is a sympathomimetic that also depresses the appetite. Many abusers of cocaine tend to be underweight and, unlike amphetamine users, they are often dehydrated, especially when cocaine use is combined with alcohol and marijuana abuse.[9]

Because of decreased carbohydrate ingestion, almost all cocaine addicts eventually suffer from ketosis. As muscle mass atrophies, amino acids are released for conversion to glucose and ketones. As the concentration of ketones rises (ketosis), it creates an excess in the urine (ketonuria) and in the blood (ketonemia). Eventually the brain begins to use ketones as fuel.

Nutritional treatment for the cocaine abuser involves a high-calorie, complex-carbohydrate diet. The complex carbohydrates are needed to reverse ketosis and provide fuel. The body will use carbohydrate as fuel before other nutrients. A vitamin and mineral supplement should be taken each day. This is quite necessary when the individual increases caloric intake.[9]

Three to four days after the body is cleared of all traces of cocaine, vitamin C supplementation should begin. The patient should have 1000 mg. of vitamin C in the morning and 1000 mg. of vitamin C in the evening. The importance of vitamin C in the cocaine withdrawal process is crucial. Not only is vitamin C a powerful aid in rebuilding nutritional status, but it is also an excellent aid in detoxification. It helps to clear the body of any residual substance. It can also eliminate or modify many of the withdrawal symptoms associated with addicting substances.[4,10,11]

The patient should also take one B-complex vitamin in the morning and one in the evening. Many heavy cocaine abusers have said they craved peanut butter at times. This is linked to the body's need for B vitamins. The patient should receive 500 mg. of B-complex three times daily and 500 mg. of pantothenic acid every day. This will aid the body in replenishing acetylcholine and other neurotransmitter levels.

Choline supplements can help to improve memory and also to treat neural and muscular problems. Although not considered as essential nutrient under normal circumstances, choline and pantothenic acid are considered essential at times of extreme stress. Recovering from cocaine abuse certainly falls into this category. Those who have repeatedly free-based cocaine will need higher dosages.[5]

Finally, our hundred I.U.'s of vitamin E every day may provide a preventative measure against circulatory and heart disease.[12]

Because of the quick absorption and elimination of cocaine, there is no effect on the gastrointestinal tract.

OPIATES

In the early stages of heroin and morphine addiction, the appetite is increased. This phase is short-lived. The abuser quickly replaces the desire to eat with the desire to use. Most hard-core heroin addicts live only to get high and eat very little, subsisting on sweets when they do eat.[10] Digestion is affected by narcotic abuse. Gastric secretions are reduced, thus reducing gastric enzyme activity, especially proteolytic.

Withdrawal from opiates is very uncomfortable. The abusers suffer gastrointestinal bleeding, hypermotility, gastrointestinal cramps, nausea, vomiting and severe tremors. This usually lasts between 2 to 5 days. Vitamin C is used to help detoxify and clear the body, as well as to help relieve some of the withdrawal symptoms. The usual treatment is 8 grams every day during the first week. This is followed by 4 to 8 grams of vitamin C orally, every 2 to 4 hours for 5 days.[5,13]

Intravenous dextrose, or large amounts of candy or pastries such as baklava, can reduce withdrawal symptoms to some degree.

Weight gain is usually a priority. Heroin addicts in recovery need to eat a protein-rich diet high in B-complex vitamins. At least 60 percent of total caloric consumption should be derived from carbohydrates. This diet will maintain serum glucose levels and raise energy output. During withdrawal, if the patient seems especially nervous or agitated, additional mineral supplements such as 1000 mg. of calcium, 90 mg. of magnesium, and 30 mg. of potassium, all given three times each day, will reduce anxiety symptoms.

STEROIDS

Anabolic steroids are often abused because of the widespread belief that they boost athletic performance. These steroids are manmade variants of testosterone.

Steroids impair the activation of vitamin D, thus negatively affecting calcium levels. Steroids also decrease the absorption of phosphorus, adding to the loss of calcium. The rate of potassium excretion is increased through steroid use. In addition, mobilization of lipids can increase the risk of coronary artery disease.

To nutritionally help the steroid abuser, a diet should be prescribed according to the individual's needs. Increasing foods rich in calcium, potassium, and vitamin D is necessary. Foods richest in potassium include apricots, bananas, cantaloupe, dates, figs, green peppers, oysters, peaches, prunes, raisins, tomatoes, peanut butter, potatoes and orange juice. Vitamin D can be obtained through consumption of milk, oysters, fish, cheese, and margarine. Dairy foods, citrus fruits, legumes, sardines, shellfish and green vegetables are all sources of calcium.[14]

CONCLUSION

Having the knowledge of proper nutrition and diet therapy is essential to aid in the healing process as a person recovers from an illness. Recovery from drug and alcohol abuse often begins with increasing the proper foods and vitamins, although each person must be evaluated individually. A dietician is a valuable member of the drug treatment team.

NOTES

1. Claydon P. Self-reported alcohol, drug and eating disorder problems of collegiate children of alcoholics. J Am Coll Health 1987; **36**:111-116.
2. Simko MD, Davidson R. Nutrition Assessment. Rockville: Aspen Publishers, 1984.

3. Dual dependency appears more difficult to treat than alcoholism. (Adapted from Addictive Behaviors 1991; **1(19)**:105-112). Brown Univ Dig Addict Theory Applic 1994; **12(2)**:8.
4. Scheer JF. Vitamin C: slice and supplement. Better Nutrition for Today's Living 1995; **57**:52
5. Mertz W. A balanced approach to nutrition for health: the need for biologically essential minerals and vitamins. J Am Dietetic Assoc (Nov) 1994; **94**:1259.
6. Langer S. Immunity building blocks: nutritional deficiencies lead to collapse. Better Nutrition for Today's Living. 1995; **57**:52.
7. Giannini AJ. (Research in progress.)
8. Giannini AJ. Drug abuse and depression: possible models for geriatric anorexia. Neurobiol Aging 1988; **9(10)**:26-27.
9. Giannini AJ. Drug abuse and depression: catecholamine depletion suggested as biological tie between cocaine withdrawal and depression. Natl Inst Drug Abuse Notes 1982; **2(2)**:5.
10. Smith, T. How dangerous is heroin? Brit Med J 1993; **307**:807.
11. Giannini AJ. Ascorbic acid and dopamine activity. Am J Psychiatry 1988; **145**;905-906.
12. Sundstrom H, Korpela H, Viinikka L, Kaupell A. Plasma liquid peroxidases and their response as antioxidants. Cancer 1984; **1(1)**:1-10.
13. Giannini AJ, Slaby AE. The Eating Disorders. New York:Springer-Verlag, 1993.
14. Leach RV. Anabolic steroids-round 4. Am J Sports Medicine 1993; **21**:337.

CHAPTER 20

LEGAL ISSUES IN DRUG ABUSE

For healthcare professionals, treating drug abuse is a matter of individual and societal well-being. While it is also a matter of well-being for the legal profession, the focus is not on the effects drug abuse has on the health of the biological system, but the effects drug abuse has on the safety of society. The legal profession thus has a slightly different interest in drug abuse than does the health profession.

The key concept of the legal approach is that of "diminished capacity." Diminished capacity refers to the user's inability to make decisions or execute actions that could reasonably be expected of an unimpaired individual. The legal focus of diminished capacity is upon restricted legal activities (e.g., driving, boating, and using firearms) and illegal activities. Impairment in the execution of restricted activities can create a situation in which property or persons are placed in danger. Diminished capacity in illegal activity can create mitigating circumstances as interpreted by a jury reaching a verdict or a judge passing sentence.[1]

RESTRICTED ACTIVITY

Any activity in which poor execution of that activity can create a danger for persons or property is considered a restricted activity. Examples include transportation and safety-sensitive areas.

All aspects of the transportation industry are covered by the restricted activity rule,[2] including restricted use of driving private cars, trucks, trains, planes and commercial shipping vehicles. In the United States, it is generally accepted that the mere operation of a land or water vehicle under the influence of alcohol or psychoactive drugs is an illegal act and it is usually defined as a misdemeanor. Commission of an illegal activity, or the production of injury to another person while under the influence, creates both criminal liability and civil liability. Depending on the jurisdiction, the amount of damage involved, and the question of personal injury to another person, the defendant may be charged with either a misdemeanor or a felony.

In the transportation industry, drug testing can be performed in most jurisdictions without cause because of the increased sensitivity of this particular activity. As a result of the 1989 U.S. Supreme Court decision in National Treasury Employees Union vs. von Raab, drug testing can be used as a screen whenever a drug-related performance danger has been clearly demonstrated.[3]

In other restricted activities, the drug screening role may not be applicable, according to the von Raab decision.[4] However, if it can be demonstrated that a dangerous situation was created by a person under the influence of drugs or alcohol, a situation of implied civil and or criminal liability is created. A surgeon who botches an operation and was shown to be under the influence of alcohol or another drug can be charged with reckless endangerment. If the surgery that was performed under the influence led to the death of an individual, the surgeon could be charged with manslaughter.

Negligent civil acts executed with a clear sensorium may become criminal acts if executed under the influence of drugs or alcohol. That is, a person who incurs civil liability because of his negligent act may find the charges against him increased to include *criminal* penalty because of his use of psychoactive substances. If a drug abuser commits a negligent act which endangers himself while in the employ of another, he may be precluded from suing for damages. For example, an individual who operates a drill press under the influence of cocaine and subsequently puts the drill bit through his hand and suffers amputation may not sue for damages if it is shown that the negligence arose from the employee's use of cocaine. However, if the employee's drug use was known to the employer and the latter took no action to stop it, then the employer will be held negligent, and the employee could be awarded damages. Because of the liability assumed by the employer, the courts have allowed mandatory drug screening as part of the job application process, whether or not employees are in safety-sensitive positions.

The military presents a special case. In 1981, a U.S. Navy jet crashed onto the aircraft carrier U.S.S. *Nimitz* killing 14 sailors and injuring an additional 42 naval personnel. A court of inquiry determined that drug abuse was a direct cause of the crash and of the subsequent deaths and injuries. As a result, the Navy instituted mandatory drug testing for all military personnel. In a six-year period from 1980 to 1986, the number of petty officers and junior officers smoking marijuana declined from 50 percent to less than 10 percent. Within three years, the Department of Defense extended the policy of mandatory drugs testing to all military personnel including soldiers, airmen and Marines. Because the Coast Guard is part of the Treasury and not the Pentagon, the Coast Guard was not included until the late 1980's.[5]

President Ronald Reagan extended the concept of the "drug-free workplace" to cover all safety-sensitive executive-level and civil service positions through Executive Order 12584.[6] By this order, mandatory laboratory testing was instituted for all employees in safety-sensitive Federal government positions. This was quickly challenged in the courts by the National Treasury Employees Union. In the 1989 von Raab decision, the Supreme Court ruled that drug testing may be ordered if "reasonable indirect concerns for public safety or welfare exists." Under President George Bush, public support developed for mandatory drug testing in the private sector. This was an element of the drug-free workplace outlined in the White House National Drug Control Strategy published in 1989.[7]

ILLEGAL ACTIVITIES

Diminished capacity may increase the amount of legal liability incurred by the defendant. In criminal cases, if the ingestion was unknowing, it can reduce the penalty or, at times, preclude a conviction.

In a notorious 1856 case, Congressman Dan Sickles murdered Philip Barton Key, the son of Francis Scott Key. The younger Key had been Sickles' wife's lover. Congressman Sickles' defense attorney was Edwin Stanton, who at that time was U.S. Attorney General and was soon to be Lincoln's Secretary of War. Because of the cast of characters, this case generated considerable excitement. Since many members of the Senate, Congress and the White House directly and indirectly participated and interfered in the trial, it was indeed "the case of the century." From this colorful and media-accentuated legal event, the concept of "temporary insanity" was developed. In this case, Sickles was deemed "temporarily insane" during the time interval in which he repeatedly shot Key while the victim begged for his life. He was considered "sane" immediately prior to and subsequent to the event.[8]

Although the temporary insanity plea may be considered an element of diminished capacity, it generally does not have universal applicability. In most cases, the knowing use of licit or illicit drugs for purposes of inducing an intoxicating state does not reduce the criminal's culpability. For example, a defendant who wounds another person under the influence of phencyclidine could not use diminished capacity as a defense. The only exception would be if he had been unknowingly supplied this drug and thus was an innocent victim of a prank with dangerous consequences.[9]

Likewise, the substance abuser who knowingly abuses a legal substance (such as Ritalin) and under its influence commits a robbery in which another person is harmed, cannot claim diminished capacity. Again, an exception would occur if the Ritalin was prescribed, the patient took it as prescribed, and was not made aware of the possibility of rage reactions, irritability or psychosis.[10] Unintentional drug abuse, or the taking of a legal drug as prescribed by a physician with unintended side effects, can be considered an offshoot of the temporary insanity law.

While some drugs can produce a verdict of "not guilty by reason of insanity," this is a rare occurrence. The insanity plea in non-drug abuse cases accounts for less than 0.2 percent of all Federal verdicts.[11] Generally, those individuals with chronic rather than organic brain damage as a result of voluntary chronic misuse of substances such as alcohol may successfully plead "insanity." If brain damage is due to alcoholic-induced pellagra or alcoholic-induced Wernicke-Korsakoff, and it causes a patient to be unable to understand the nature of his crime, or to refrain from committing his crime, or if it renders him unable to understand the consequences of his crime, a plea of "insanity" may be entered.[12] Furthermore, if, due to the long-time use of drugs or because of unintended permanent effects of the drug (e.g., cerebral vascular accident caused by a single use of a volatile agent), the person may be judged incompetent to stand trial. These are patients who cannot understand the nature of the trial or cannot participate meaningfully in their defense.[13] In this case, the offender may be confined to a criminal hospital.

Hospitalization will be continued only in the likelihood that competency can be achieved in a reasonable amount of time. The reasonable time interval is determined by the legal system. If the time duration is judged not to be reasonable, three alternatives to criminal hospital status are available. The defendant who is incompetent to stand trial may be given a trial with special protections developed by the court, or the defendant may be civilly committed to an institution as mentally ill or, in unusual cases, the defendant may be released and the criminal charges erased.[1]

DRIVING UNDER THE INFLUENCE

Alcoholic impairment while operating a motor vehicle is an important issue. Approximately one-half of all fatally injured drivers have been determined to have been drinking alcohol a short period prior to their driving. In the 25 to 65 age group, between 60 to 75 percent of all fatalities involve alcohol.[14]

On the highways, most states allow police officers to examine for alcohol intoxication any person who is speeding, driving in an erratic manner or has been involved in an accident. In addition, most states and territories within the United States permit random inspection of drivers, especially during the holidays, which are associated with higher motor vehicle fatality rates.

The presence of alcohol alone, however, is not *legally* considered to be proof of impairment. A physiological concentration of 0.06 to 0.10 percent is considered to be over the maximum permitted.[15] Depending upon the state, drivers in excess of these levels are considered "driving under the influence" or "driving while intoxicated" (DUI or DWI).

Alcohol intoxication usually is determined by using the "breathalizer" test. In many states, if the driver is found to be intoxicated while operating a motor vehicle, his license is suspended until his trial. Also, if the driver refuses to be tested by a breathalizer or serum blood test, this is considered proof of guilt.

With either laboratory confirmation or presumed proof of guilt, the legal result is the same. Sanctions usually involve loss of license for a period of time, enforced attendance in alcohol treatment programs, a fine, and publication of the driver's name or some other sanction for the first offense. Later offenses can bring permanent loss of the driver's license or impoundment of his or her motor vehicle.

Recently, there have been several legal challenges to the above practice. Intoxicated drivers have argued that they are unfairly placed in a position of "double jeopardy" by the loss of license and a subsequent court hearing (note: double jeopardy refers to being tried twice for the same offense). Lower courts have agreed with the defendants' argument. This legal practice is under appeal and its resolution is uncertain.

Alcoholics who are frequently arrested for operating a motor vehicle when drunk may find themselves civilly committed under the Uniform Alcoholism and Intoxication Treatment Act. This act, which has been adopted by a majority of states, is used to force alcoholics into treatment programs by encouraging voluntary treatment or, utilizing civil commitment, by forcing involuntary treatment. Under this act, an alcoholic is defined as any person who uses alcohol "...to the extent that his health is substantially impaired or endangered or his socioeconomic function is substantially disrupted." Furthermore, involuntary commitment is allowed only if the alcohol creates cognitive deficiencies or confusion.

NOTES

1. Gunn J, Taylor PJ. Forensic Psychiatry: Clinical, Legal and Ethical issues. Stonecham, Mass: Butterworth-Heinemann, 1993.
2. Skinner vs. Railway Labor Executives Association. 1984; 87-1555 (US Supreme Court).
3. National Treasury Employer's Union vs. von Raab, 1989; 86-1879.
4. Nelkin D, Tancredi LR. Dangerous Diagnostics. New York: Basic Books, 1989.
5. Miller NS, Giannini AJ, Gold MS, Philomena JA. Drug testing: medical, legal and ethical issues. J Substance Abuse Treatment 1990; 7:239-244.
6. Presidential Documents. Executive Order 12584. Federal Register 1986; **51**:180.
7. White House National Drug Control Strategy. Washington DC, US Govt Printing Office, 1989.
8. Swanberg WA. Sickles the Incredible. Gettysburg, PA: S.C. Military Books, 1991.
9. Ohio vs. Burke C-184, 1980.
10. Tancredi LR, Giannini AJ. The admissability of scientific evidence in psychiatric malpractice. J Clin Forensic Med (Great Britain) 1994; **1**:145-149.
11. Dershowitz AM. Abolishing the insanity defense. Crim Law Bull 1973; **9**:434-439.

12. Scott PD. The Butler Committees report: psychiatric aspects. Br J Criminal 1976; **16**:177-178.
13. U.S. vs. Brawner, 471 F. 2d. 969, DC Cir, 1972.
14. Alcohol and Health. First Special Report to the US Congress from the Secretary of HEW, Natl Inst of Alcohol Abuse and Alcoholism. Washington, DC, 1971.
15. Perrine MW. Alcohol, drugs and driving. Proc Sixth Int Conf Alcohol Drugs Traffic Safety Sept 8-13, 1974.

CHAPTER 21

DRUG TESTING

In the field of chemical dependency, laboratory testing serves multiple purposes. As in other fields of medicine, the clinical laboratory can assist in confirming a diagnosis. Lab testing can also be used for nonmedical purposes, such as determining feasibility for employment, criminal culpability, and liability in court cases. Ordering a drug test has legal and ethical, as well as medical, implications.[1]

Physicians who have traditionally embraced diagnostic testing procedures, however, have been slow to adopt drug testing. Perhaps this is because physicians generally rely on patient cooperation and compliance for their diagnostic test. Drug testing generally deals with a patient population that often denies the disease of addiction and resists the therapeutic modification offered by the physician.[2]

LEGAL ISSUES

Generally, drug testing can be performed anytime, upon any person in the United States as long as an explicit or implicit agreement exists between the test-giver and the test-taker.[1] When such an agreement does not exist, drug testing may be imposed. Most states allow on-site drug and alcohol testing upon reasonable suspicion by a police officer. The Supreme Court ruled in 1989 in the National Treasury Employees Union vs. von Raab that testing may be imposed wherever there is reasonable risk of injury or impairment of performance which may render an employee a danger to himself or others.[3] Drug testing can also be imposed, according to the Supreme Court, in the transportation industry (Skinner vs. Railway Labor Executive's Association, 1989).[4]

Indeed, employers who operate car fleets, truck fleets, trains, planes, buses, and commercial shipping vessels are required to periodically test their employees. Also, most attorney generals and county prosecutors have interpreted the von Raab decision to mean that drug testing may be ordered where reasonable and direct concerns for public safety or welfare exist.

However, as a result of the von Raab decision, employers are precluded from utilizing drug screens where drug-related performance danger has not been clearly demonstrated. Drug testing, however, may be used as an element of the initial job interview. While this has not been fully tested by the Supreme Court, it has been supported by the White House through Executive Order 12584 in 1986.[5] It received further executive support upon publication of the White House National Drug Control Strategy in 1989.[6]

DRUG TESTING METHODOLOGY

The target of drug testing can either be the drug itself or one of its metabolites. The samples can be obtained from either the blood or the urine. In most situations, urine is the ideal sample source due to the concentrating effects of the kidneys.

Urine contains 100 to 1000 times more of the drug or its metabolite than serum samples.[5] Serum samples, however, can be used to determine time of ingestion. Each drug has a specific time before it is biotransformed and eliminated. Therefore, testing of both serum and urine levels can determine, with reasonable accuracy, the approximate time of ingestion. In cases where a drug has a particularly short elimination time, however, serum levels are useless.

When ordering a specific test, sensitivity and specificity must be considered. Drug testing differs from traditional laboratory testing since the specificity, sensitivity and source of the sample must all be considered. Generally, a medical doctor will test red blood cells by ordering a CBC (complete blood test), or serum chemistry by ordering an SMAC (sequential multiple analyses, computerized), and it's not necessary for the ordering physician to specify a particular method.

Specificity is the degree of accuracy in detecting only the drug desired. If the test is highly specific, it will avoid a false positive result. For example, reacting with relatively harmless pseudoephedrine in a test for cocaine would yield a false positive result.

Sensitivity refers to the degree at which low concentrations of the specific drug may be tested. Tests with low specificity tend to have a high amount of false positives. Tests with low sensitivity tend to report a high rate of false negatives. False negative tests outnumber false positive tests by at least 10 to 1. A study of cocaine testing conducted by the Centers for Disease Control found that most laboratories have a 75 percent false negative rate.[7]

There are two major types of methodology in drug testing: chromatographic tests and immunoassay. In addition, indirect tests can be ordered which do not test for the drug or metabolite but instead examine endocrinological effects of particular drugs.[8]

CHROMATOGRAPHIC TESTING

All chromatographic tests rely upon a characteristic and reproducible migration pattern produced by a particular drug. Common chromatographic assays include thin layer chromatography (TLC), gas-liquid chromatography (GLC), high pressure liquid chromatography (HPLC), gas chromatography (GC) and mass spectrometry (MS). Chromatographic techniques generally require sample extraction with an organic solvent. After dissolving the sample, pH must be adjusted so that the drug to be tested is selectively driven into the organic solvent during the partition process. This ionization drive process concentrates the particular drug being tested. As a result, chromatographic assays are quantitatively specific at low levels of serum or urine concentration.

Thin layer chromatography (TLC) is the most commonly employed initial screen for drugs. It is a relatively fast and inexpensive test. Unfortunately, TLC does not lend itself to quantification, it is a qualitative test only. Unlike other chromatographic tests, it has very low sensitivity and low specificity. As a result of its low sensitivity, drug concentrations of less than 1000-2000 ng/ml. are read as falsely negative.

TLC plates must be read by a trained technician in a subjective manner. As a result, TLC is usually not acceptable by the legal system. In performing the TLC, the ionized sample is generally placed on a silica coated glass plate (i.e., the "thin layer"). The drug is allowed to migrate and then is detected by spraying the glass plate with a color-complexing reagent. The technician generally will view the migration pattern and subjectively identity the drug in this particular sample.

Greater specificity is achieved by gas-liquid chromatography (GLC). In utilizing GLC, molecules are separated by a glass tube packed with polarized material. The sample within the tube is then vaporized after being injected into the chromatographic apparatus and carried through a column by gas flow. The time required to pass though the column is referred to as the retention time. Each drug has a unique retention time in a given column. After passing through the column, the sample comes in contact with the detector that reports and quantifies the drug or drugs present. High pressure liquid chromatography (HPLC) is similar to GLC except that liquid rather than gas is used to propel the testing sample through the column.

IMMUNOLOGIC ASSAY TESTS

Immunologic assays are derived from the immune response between a particular drug and a specific antibody. These antibodies are derived from animal serum. They are mixed with a serum or urine sample from the patient, and the number of binding sites is measured by enzymatic, fluorescent or radioactive tagging. By this determination, the ratio of free to bound antibody at equilibrium can be determined.

The type of tag employed determines the test. Enzyme tagging produces the enzyme immunoassay (EIA); fluorescent tagging, the fluorescent polarization immunoassay (FPIA); and radioactive isotope tagging, radioactive isotope immunoassay (RIA).

Glucose-6-phosphate dehydrogenase (G6PD) is the tag used in EIA. With this tag, the reduction of NAD to NADH can be measured on a spectrophotometer at a wave length of 340 Nm. Fluorescent polarization uses a fluorescent tag to measure the ratio of bound to unbound antibodies. In RIA, radioactive iodine (I^{125}) is the most commonly employed tag. In this test, the greater the concentration of drug, the greater the amount of free radioactive antigen and solution producing a higher degree of radioactivity which can be measured in a scintillation counter.

In immunoassays, false positives and falsely elevated results can be produced by cross-reactivity of the antibodies. The sensitivity of the test also is dependent upon the actual antibodies employed. Immunoassays, although much more sensitive than chromatographic techniques, are not as specific as gas-liquid chromatography or mass spectrometry.

APPLICATIONS IN THE REAL WORLD

Since each testing procedure has its relative merits and demerits, most direct-testing protocols utilize a combination of chromatography and immunoassay. An inpatient unit generally uses first-morning urine samples, whereas outpatient centers rely upon random sampling.

Generally, the patient voids under supervision to avoid tampering by dilution or substitution. A commonly employed safeguard is temperature measurement. Urine samples which are not at or near body temperature are assumed to have been diluted or substituted. If temperature measurement is not possible, specific gravity and pH can be tested to rule out dilution. These latter techniques will not, however, detect a substitution. First-morning urine sampling is a preferred technique because of the relatively high level of concentration in a relatively large volume of fluid.

In the emergency room, when the question of recent drug ingestion is posed, serum levels are preferred to urine. Because of relatively high rates of metabolism for most drugs of abuse, serum samples can determine recent ingestion. It can also determine which patients were under the influence for legal purposes.[9]

The initial sample can be performed by automated EIA or RIA. These assays have a high level of sensitivity. Negative assays can be presumed to establish that a patient is drug-free or has not abused drugs in the time interval determined by specific drug metabolism. Unfortunately, immunoassays are not particularly sensitive so positive assay may be the result of a true positive or false positive. When immunoassay is found to be positive, GS/MS confirms the accuracy or inaccuracy of immunoassay positive results.

NOTES

1. Nelkin DN, Tancredi LR. Dangerous Diagnostics. New York: Basic Books, 1989.
2. Stark M. Working with Resistance. New York: Jason Aronson, 1994.
3. National Treasury Employee's Union vs. von Raab. 86-1879, U.S. Supreme Court, 1989.
4. Skinner vs. Railway Labor Executives Association 87-15555, U.S. Supreme Court, 1989.
5. Presidential Documents. Executive Order 12584. Federal Register **51**:L180,1986.
6. White House National Drug Control Strategy. Washington DC: US Government Printing Office, 1984.
7. Hansen HJ, Cardill SP, Boone DJ. Crisis in drug testing: results of the CDC blind study. JAMA 1985; **25**:2382-2387.

8. Miller NS, Giannini AJ, Gold MS, Philomena JA. Drug testing: medical, legal and ethical issues. J Substance Abuse Treatment 1990; **7**:239-244.

9. Calderoaro G. Eroina, mercato al consumo é ruolo delle organizzazoni criminals. VII Seminario Nazionale per Professori, Italiani di Discipline Criminaloqiche. Syracuse, Italy, October 12-14, 1989.

CHAPTER 22

ORGANIZATION OF ADDICTION UNITS

There are numerous and sometimes divergent schools of thought about the best treatment modalities involved in drug therapy. All the different models, however, can be reduced to two basic types. These are the "pure" inpatient treatment unit, and the hybrid inpatient detoxification/outpatient rehabilitation model. In the former model, all detoxification and rehabilitation takes place within the confines of an inpatient unit. Confining the patient to this unit for treatment removes him or her from the pressures and temptations of the outside world. In the latter model, only detoxification is done on an inpatient basis. The patient is discharged and attends an outpatient treatment center while he or she continues to live at home. Both models involve the removal of the drug from the patient and the reduction of the reinforcers to continue drug use.[1]

Some drugs, such as marijuana, are very easy to detoxify and do not require much medical support. However, others, such as the barbiturates, involve a withdrawal process which can be life threatening (see Table 22-1).

There are multiple reinforcers to continue drug use. Primary reinforcers include the euphoria it offers and the cravings of the withdrawal state. The euphoria is considered a positive reinforcer since it produces a highly pleasurable sensation. The unpleasant cravings and symptoms associated with drug withdrawal are negative reinforcers. The drug withdrawal state, as with all negative reinforcers, is a state to be avoided. The only common path of avoidance for the addict is the continued abuse of the drug to which he or she is addicted.[2]

In addition to primary reinforcers, there are five common secondary reinforcers. These include visual, environmental, social, activity and intrapsychic reinforcers. Each secondary reinforcer acts as a trigger which can set off a craving for a particular drug. Visual triggers include sight recognition of those objects commonly associated with the drug state.

Table 22-1: Guide to Inpatient Detoxification

Drug	Detoxicant Drug	Post-Detox Protocol	Special Interventions	Avg. Days Detox
Alcohol	Chlordiaze-poxide	Nutritional maintenance (use thiamine, folic acid, magnesium)	Seizure precautions	3-4
Amphetamine	Bromocriptine	Desipramine, nutritional maintenance	None	4-6
Anticholin-ergics (high dose only)	Physostigmine salicylate	None	Seizure precautions, monitor possible ileus, atonic bladder & cardiac status monitoring, rehydrate, maintain blood pressure	2-3
Benzodiaze-pines	Any benzodiazepine	Hydroxyzine or beta-blocker	Seizure precautions	3-4
Cocaine	Bromocriptine	Desipramine, nutritional maintenance	Nutritional maintenance, cardiac monitoring for possible cocaethylene induced complications	4-6
Khat	Bromocriptine	Desipramine	None	3-4
Opiates	Clonidine	Trazodone or methadone	Bed rest, monitor blood pressure	3-5
Phencyclidine	Haloperidol	Desipramine	Possible restraints, precautions for violence, acidify urine	1-2
Psychedelics	Hydroxyzine or benzodiazepine	Fluoxetine	Minimal environmental stimulation	1/2-2
Sedative-hypnotics	Phenobarbital	—	Seizure precautions, maintain blood pressure, cardiac monitoring, treat acidosis, treat hypothermia	3-6
Steroids	None	Nutritional maintenance, antipsychotics & antidepressents, prn	Rigorous physical therapy, NSAID's for muscular pain, precautions for violence, possible cardiac monitoring	1-3
Volatiles	None	Neuroleptics, prn	Investigate possible hepatic, bone marrow, & peripheral & neurological pathologies	1-3

Because of this, a cocaine addict's craving may reappear after he or she sees white powder or paraphernalia, such as mirrors or razor blades, which are associated with the drug usage. Environmental triggers can include the surroundings which were associated with the drug-abusing state. Examples include the heroin addict who returns to his or her neighborhood where previously the addict was able to easily purchase the heroin. The camaraderie of a neighborhood bar may be a social trigger which reignites a craving for alcohol. Weight lifting can be thought of as an activity trigger which creates a sense of addiction in a steroid addict. Intrapsychic triggers include a sense of achievement or status associated respectively with marijuana or amphetamine use.[3]

In both models, the patient is treated with a team approach. Although the components of the team may vary among institutions, a team almost always includes a psychiatrist who performs the actual evaluation and detoxification, an internist who deals with severe medical complications, and registered nurses or possibly licensed practical nurses who perform nursing and counseling duties. Usually there are certified alcohol counselors or certified addiction counselors who, in many cases, are recovering addicts. These key members of the team provide support and a practical counseling approach.

Many units also utilize other specialists. These include licensed social workers to deal with the social, familial, neighborhood, and vocational environments of the addict. Registered dieticians or nutritional counselors are important partners of some teams and provide the patients with methods to maintain their own good health. Occupational therapists generally emphasize a system which leads to the acquisition of life skills that can promote increased competency and a sense of achievement.

The ultimate goal in any model utilized is to move the patient from a dependent role to an independent one. Usually the intermediate step of interdependence is utilized. This interdependence is fostered between the patient, other patient members on the unit, and the treatment team. During and after discharge, this interdependence is fostered by members of the various "anonymous" groups, such as Alcoholics Anonymous, Narcotics Anonymous and Cocaine Anonymous.[4]

When the patient is admitted, the intake process always includes a comprehensive psychiatric and medical evaluation. This is generally followed by family and environmental profiles.

After being admitted, the patient usually signs a contract to obey the unit rules. Generally, these unit rules involve abstinence clauses, search and seizure clauses, and gateway clauses. Likewise, family members are subject to staff restrictions and stated unit rules.

Gateway rules usually restrict the patient's exit and re-entry to the unit, as well as the entry and exit by family or friends. He or she usually must stay on the unit unless certain rules are met and permission to leave is given by the staff. Search and seizure powers invested in the staff allow them to perform random or scheduled drug screens, and to search the patient's body and belongings for the presence of drugs or drug paraphernalia. In addition, many units interpret the search and seizure rule as implied permission to test for HIV, hepatitis A and B antigens, and any other infectious diseases that may prove dangerous to the patient, other patients, or staff. Abstinence rules include not only refraining from various drugs of abuse, but also from sexual activity with other members of the patient group. Telephone privileges generally come under both the abstinence rules and the gateway rules. The staff restricts the type of telephone calls as well as the frequency and duration.

The immediate post-admission goals are detoxification and simultaneous sequestration from the drug-abusing environment. After these initial goals are met, the patient is assisted in his ability to utilize positive supportive elements, such as the treatment team and the various "anonymous" groups. As the patient continues to develop, moving from dependency to independence, the patient should increase his or her ability to make competent goal-directed, growth-oriented decisions. As healthy, adaptive behavior is developed, the patient is able to reduce the effects of his previous incapacity and restructure his daily living patterns. Finally, the patient will be able to eliminate most of the negative elements in his life environment; reduce the influence of those elements that cannot be eliminated (e.g., physical and intellectual limitations); and engineer healthy developments (such as a new job, new neighborhood, new job, or new friends).[5]

INPATIENT MODEL

The more traditional model involves a continuum of services rendered exclusively in an inpatient mode. The site is usually located in a general psychiatric hospital. Therapy occurs in a designated unit which provides only drug detoxification and rehabilitation services. The patient is detoxified here or, alternatively, detoxified elsewhere in the hospital but is brought to the unit to participate in some programs. As detoxification proceeds or is completed, the patient may then be transferred to the unit full-time to participate in all of its services.[6,7]

Since the unit is usually located in a hospital, the staff will include an internist who will work as a consultant for medical complications associated with the detoxification protocol. The internist may also treat related medical problems, such as hepatitis, or unrelated medical problems, such as diabetes, which may compound the detoxification or rehabilitation process. Since the model is usually hospital-based or related, registered nurses (RN) or licensed practical nurses (LPN) are utilized to monitor medication and vital signs, to routinely assess the patient's general medical progress, to report on the patient's activity or status, and, sometimes, to provide counseling.

A psychiatrist provides administrative medical services as well as detoxification psychotherapeutic services. Individual therapy is given by the psychiatrist although he or she may utilize other psychiatrists or psychologists for this purpose. Group therapy or group counseling is usually provided by the psychiatrist although other professionals can be utilized. Certified chemical dependency counselors (CCDC) or certified alcohol counselors (CAC) provide ongoing counseling. AA, NA and CA meetings are held directly on the unit to initiate a bridge between the isolated milieu of the inpatient unit and the "outside" world.

Licensed social workers (LSW, LISW or MSW) usually interact with the family, employer, social services agency or the courts. Registered dieticians (RD) and nutritionists provide dietary plans and, in many units, ongoing nutritional counseling. Some units utilize activity therapists (AT), occupational therapists (OT) or art therapists to enhance the treatment program.

A variety of treatment processes are available. Generally, detoxification is the initial modality and is supplemented by general medical maintenance. Counseling and therapy from a variety of sources, including a psychiatrist, a psychologist, the nursing staff, drug counselors and an occupational therapist, are utilized to assist the patient in learning, relearning and modifying life skills to enhance the decision-making process. Generally, the occupational therapist works with the family, the social worker and the dietician, while taking direction from the chief psychiatrist. Family therapy is usually conducted by the social workers, although the psychiatrist may involve himself or herself in this process. The nutritionist generally works with the occupational therapist in maintaining adaptive life behavior.

Group therapy enhances the interdependent and adaptive process. Interpersonal and intrapsychic conflicts are generally handled by the psychiatrist or psychologist in group therapy. Family group therapy with or without the patient's presence is generally conducted by the licensed social worker. Task-oriented therapy is generally offered by the occupational therapists. Discussion of ongoing problems with the family or within the unit itself is generally under the direction of the nursing staff.

Embracing all of these therapeutic modalities is the "therapeutic milieu." The therapeutic milieu integrates all of the above by the team-approach in which patients can interact and can provide input to the treatment team in a structured or unstructured setting. Many units use a token economy in which mastery of certain skills is rewarded with specific privileges. Each privilege level involves a greater degree of trust and independence.[2,3]

The length of stay on the unit is generally predetermined. It generally ranges from 21 to 30 days. The addict is expected to achieve certain milestones in a timely fashion. The time commitment is generally semipermeable. The addict is seldom discharged before the time interval is up. And the staff may extend the treatment process if it is felt that the addict has had supervening factors which have interfered with his therapy and that he is acting in good faith.

INPATIENT DETOX/OUTPATIENT REHAB MODEL

This model usually involves treatment being rendered at two sites. The initial detoxification is done in a hospital inpatient setting, but rehabilitation is done strictly on an outpatient basis.

In this model, detoxification is conducted by a psychiatrist or internist in a general hospital. Within the hospital, the site may involve a designated detoxification unit or a subunit of a general medical surgical floor. In either case, the staff is limited to the detoxifying physician, either an internist or psychiatrist, and a specially trained nursing staff.

A third type of unit, recently conceived in an era of declining finances, is an organizational rather than physical construct. In this third type, beds are assigned throughout the hospital on a space-available basis. General nursing or supportive services are provided by the staff on the units to which the patients are assigned. Medical detoxification, however, is rendered by the designated physician. Nursing personnel who are members of the detoxification team are assigned as liaisons to the nursing staff on the particular floors. The chemical dependency nurses in this latter model provide advice and support in specific areas of detoxification, interpretation of symptoms, general education, guidance in dealing with manipulative patients, and maintenance of boundaries. These boundaries include limitations on visitors and enforcement of search and seizure rules.[8]

The length of stay on the medical detoxification unit is usually quite short (see Table 22-1). Generally, the physician works with a predetermined protocol using detoxicant substances. The team approach is generally not strong here. The physician makes the decisions and is under no peer pressure to consult with members of the team.

In an inpatient detoxification unit, the focus is on a reduction of symptoms associated with the withdrawal state and the treatment of any complications which may ensue. Patients are confined to their bed or room. Psychotherapy and counseling is not rendered.

Dietary intervention is limited to planning a diet during the treatment program, and is generally limited to treating nutritional deficiencies which are usually associated with the drug-dependent state. Examples include a high magnesium diet in the case of alcoholics, or an American Diabetic Association diet in the case of addicts who are diabetic.

The detoxification unit, however, can be modified. Many programs utilize a contact person from the affiliated outpatient unit to introduce their programs to the patient and maintain contact until the patient is discharged. Some programs, especially those in Europe, utilize a drop-in center on the unit. This is generally a room in which ambulatory patients may, at the physician's discretion, visit during designated hours to interact with other patients. Sometimes this informal process is strengthened by a daily group therapy session at the drop-in center.[9]

After detoxification, the patient is usually discharged to an outpatient rehabilitation center. Sometimes the patient is conveyed by members of the hospital staff. Other times it is the patient's own responsibility to attend the initial session. The center may be located within the hospital or may exist as a free-standing site.

Staffing at the center is usually nonmedical and includes a social worker, certified drug counselors and possibly a registered nurse. Most centers have a psychiatrist on-call for medical emergencies and to facilitate inpatient detoxification admissions for relapsing patients. This physician is generally not based at the center.

The program is usually time-limited. It generally lasts from four to six hours per day, and it is scheduled four to five days per week. While a few programs are open-ended, most have a finite duration of four to five weeks.

After graduation, all outpatient programs refer their patients to Alcoholics Anonymous, Narcotics Anonymous, or Cocaine Anonymous, etc. Some outpatient rehabilitation units maintain an "alumni program." In this program, recovering addicts who have graduated from the center attend weekly or biweekly sessions lasting one to two hours. Sometimes these sessions include family members. These programs may be time-limited or proceed for an indefinite period according to the philosophy of the program.

Outpatient programs are generally organized around the 12-step model and involve development of group identity to facilitate the interdependent process. There is generally individual counseling which is provided by counselors who are usually recovering addicts. There is also individual therapy to deal with unique problems of the particular addict. Family therapy and group therapy are generally organized around a group treatment process. Some programs provide nutritional counseling and psychiatric occupational therapy but, usually, most programs are too small or financially limited to provide these services.

Although the outpatient treatment model is preferred by many insurance companies, its initial foundation was not economic. This model was constructed as a reaction against inpatient rehabilitation models. Founders of this type of treatment program felt that real recovery could not take place in isolation. Their point of view was that "anyone could stay drug-free on an island." Rehabilitation could not take place unless the patient interacted during his recovery process with those elements in his environment that provoked and maintained his drug-seeking behavior.[10]

In the resultant outpatient rehabilitation programs, addicts are encouraged to interact with elements of their environment that can not be changed. As a result, they are able to bring the current emotional state and problems to the staff and peer group for immediate consultation and intervention.

Immediate return to work is strongly encouraged and may be a prerequisite for admission into these units. Being productive as a worker or student is seen as a method of maintaining a sense of self-esteem and diminishing the probability of a dependency posture re-emerging.

The addict is usually required to move back with the family. By maintaining active membership in the family structure while undergoing rehabilitation, he is able to bring the members of his family into the active treatment process, facilitate family therapy and reduce co-dependency.[11]

CONCLUSION

Both treatment models have approximately equal rates of success. The selection of the particular model may be based on community resources, the physician's knowledge, the patient's need and, ever more likely, the patient's health insurance or managed care program.

The treating physician should make herself or himself thoroughly familiar with both concepts. In this manner, the patient's treatment options are maximized. The addict can then be directed to that program which most suits his or her needs. By thoroughly understanding each of the programs, the treating physician can make the appropriate referral.

NOTES

1. Cheek FE, Laucius J. The time works of three drug using groups—alcoholics, heroin addicts and psychedelics. In: Yaker HM, Osmond H, Cheek F. (Eds.), The Future of Time. New York: Doubleday, 1976.
2. Rotter J. Generalized expectancies for internal versus external control of reinforcement. Psychol Monogr 1966; **80**:1-28.
3. Huba G, Bentler P. A developmental theory of drug use: derivation and assessment of a casual modeling approach. In: Brim OG (Eds.), Life-Span Development and Behavior. New York: Academic, 1982.
4. Baekeland F. Evaluation of treatment methods in chronic alcoholism. In: Kissin B, Begleiter H. (Eds.), The Biology of Alcoholism. New York: Plenum, 1977.
5. Writh M, Obitz F. Alcoholics and nonalcoholics attribution of control of future life events. J Stud Alcohol 1984; **45**:138-143.
6. Fink A, Longbaugh R, McCrady B, et al: Effectiveness of alcoholism treatment in partial versus inpatient setting. Addict Behav 1985; **18(2)**:235-248.

7. Miller M, Gorski T, Miller D. Learning to Live Again: A Guide for Recovery from Alcoholism, 3rd ed. Missouri: Independence Press, 1982.

8. Miller RE, Giannini AJ, Gold MS, Philomena JA. Drug testing: medical, legal and ethical issues. J. Substance Abuse Treatment. 1990; **7**:239-243.

9. Giannini AJ. Hapko bn3hncot. [Note: English trans. from Macedonian: *In the Claws of the Crack Truth.*] Vecer 1990; **45(10)**:10.

10. Giannini AJ. Chemical Abuse Centers Inc.—The outpatient model of addiction recovery. Presented to the National Conference on Crack and Cocaine Addiction. Milan, Italy. January 18-20, 1990.

11. Folts DF, Giannini AJ. Cognitive workload. In: L. Jacobs & R. Betancourt (Eds.), Ergonomics for Therapists. Boston: Butterworth-Heineman, 1995.

APPENDIX A

DRUG USE AS EXPRESSED IN ART, LITERATURE AND MUSIC THROUGHOUT THE AGES

Previous chapters of this book discussed the psychiatric motivation, receptor activity, sociological impulses, hormonal secretions and cultural influences affecting individuals who abuse drugs in our society. While such chapters are a necessary part of the transmission of scientific knowledge, they lack the *gestalt* of the experience of being and treating a drug abuser.

The artist, the novelist, the historian and the film producer, who may not write or paint with perfect scientific erudition, nevertheless may reproduce accurately the sweat and fire of addiction and withdrawal. The novel, the historical analysis, the painting, the sculpture, the play and the film carry the intuitive "feel" of chemical dependency. Through the eye of the artist, we can experience the alterations of feeling and thought which accompanies the liquids and powders with which the addict alters his reality.[1]

ANCIENT HISTORY AND MYTHOLOGY

Some of the first references to mind- and mood-altering drugs are found in the book of Genesis and *The Gilgamesh Epic*. In Genesis, Noah discovers alcohol after the flood and engages in drunken foolishness. His son, Ham, laughs at him but does not intervene, and is divinely punished. In the *Gilgamesh Epic*, the hero Gilgamesh becomes drunk and loses the favor of the gods and possibly his immortality. Also in the Bible, marijuana is discussed in the Song of Songs; and Samson looses his power when he becomes drunk and has his hair shorn by Delilah in the book of Prophets.

References to alcohol and intoxicating drugs are also found in classical mythology. Greek mythology assigned a god, Dionysus (the Roman god Bacchus), to the supervision of grapes and their fermentation into wine. One myth describes wild parties in which the hero of music, Orpheus, was destroyed by the followers of Dionysus. The Greeks later developed the tradition of the sibyls: women who inhaled vapors venting from geological fissures or from the burning of various herbs. In Greek epic poems and mythology, the sibyls' hallucinations guide adventurers and kings.

In Homer's *Iliad*, Helen of Troy gives Telemachus marijuana. Later, the hero, King Ajax the Greater, dies during a drunken frenzy. Afterwards, the war hero Odysseus wanders throughout the Mediterranean for 10 years, his travels recorded in the *Odyssey*. He encounters the land of the lotus eaters, whose residents' addiction to opium threatens the integrity of his crew. Later, the crewmembers are again nearly destroyed by the psychedelic powers of the sorceress, Circe.

Viking mythology tells the story of the otherwise invincible Thor, god of thunder, who is bested by evil giants in his failure to drain a horn of mead. Alcohol and botanicals are also depicted as destructive forces in the *Aeneid*, the work of the Roman poet, Virgil.

Possibly the earliest documentation of an alcoholic beverage was found in ancient Sumerian fragments which described the recipe for making beer from barley. Greek literature later dealt with the follies of alcohol in the plays of Aristophanes. The early historian, Xenephon, discussed the destructive potential of wine in *Oeconomicus*, a sort of marital instruction manual for husbands.[2] His *Hellenic* and the histories of his contemporary Thucydides describe the deleterious effects of wine upon the Athenians and the more disciplined Spartans.

Roman historians first describe the effects of a drug which may have been khat in Gaius Sallustius Crispus' *Jugurthine Wars*.[3] Plutarch, the greatest of early Roman historians, does not mention alcohol; although the late empire historian, Dio Cassius Cocceianus, discusses the deleterious effects of alcohol, opium and marijuana in the decay of the Empire.[4] Both Greek and Roman historians refer to the use of marijuana by the ancient Hittites who defeated the armies of the Pharaoh until they were undone by their addiction to marijuana. The Neronian novelist, Titus Petronius Arbitar, describes the chemical excesses of the early days of the empire. His *Satyricon* focusses on alcoholism and bulimia, whereas *The Feast of Trimalchios* discusses abuse of alcohol, opium and, possibly, strychnine.[5]

Sumerian art shows statues which are realistic and anatomically correct except for the appearance of the eyes: all Sumerian sculptors carved greatly enlarged eye sockets. This may have been an artistic device to demonstrate dilated pupils. It would not be inconsistent with the use of sympathomimetic drugs, such as khat, or many of the atropinic drugs which grew in the region of Sumer three thousand years ago. Statues of Gudea, the semi-mythic leader, also hint at the use of sympathomimetics and anticholinergics.[6] Both Greek and the later derivative Roman statues repeatedly revisited the theme of "The Drunken Satyr." There are also statues, especially from Roman time, of Bacchus in a drunken pose. And the so-called "Pompeii murals" show men and women in various stages of drunkenness and hangover.[7]

MEDIEVAL EUROPE

With the fall of Rome, discussion of drugs of abuse shifted to the Catholic church's morality plays, where alcoholism was seen as a cardinal sin. The Holy Roman Emperor Charlemagne worried about the effects of alcohol on the fitness of his troops. Several early historians, including Alcuin of York and the Venerable Bede, penned numerous tracts reflecting societal concerns.[8]

At the birth of eleventh century, there appeared a new art form. These were the songs of the troubadours, the "Chansons," which dealt with courtly love. The first major troubadour was Duke William of Aquitaine, born in 1071. What is interesting for the drug historian is that his songs' description of unrequited love are similar to the highs and withdrawal symptoms of many drugs of abuse. These lyrics describe shivers and sweats, chills and fevers. These ecstasies of love produced periods of anesthesia as well as periods of highs and lows, confusion and hyperactivity.[9]

In counterpoint, the sermons of Bernard Clairvaux were "anti" everything, including anti-alcohol and anti-pleasure. Bernard, however, seems to have been an anorectic whose visions may be attributed to starvation ketosis or ingestion of rye infected with the fungus causing St. Anthony's fire, which is a painful psychedelic state caused by the fungus *Clavicups purpura*.[10] Many German mystics certainly suffered from St. Anthony's fire.[11] The Italian poet Dante Alighieri placed drunkards in *Purgatoreo*.[12] His fellow Florentine, Giovanni Boccaccio, however, did not share his moralistic attitude.[13] Alcohol was seen by Boccaccio as a release, enhancing life's joys and distancing one from life's travails. Boccaccio's imitator, the English poet Geoffrey Chaucer, struck a similar chord in *Canterbury Tales*.

The all-time best-seller of the Middle Ages, the *Romance of the Rose*, many times compared love to alcoholism and drunkenness.[14] This romantic interdigitation of love and alcohol was continued in the *Letters* of Abelard and Heloise. The famous philosopher Abelard and his student-cum-lover, Heloise, were a real-life Romeo and Juliet whose relationship requited, shocked, entranced, entertained and enthralled literate Europe.[15]

RENAISSANCE EUROPE AND EARLY AMERICA

During the Renaissance, alcohol, opium, marijuana and belladonna were commonly used drugs of abuse. The explorations of Columbus and the depredations of the *Conquistadors* brought cocaine and, possibly, mescaline to Europe.

Generally the Italian schools of art depicted idealized forms. In Northern Europe with its harsher climate, the darker, less-idealized side of man was depicted in visual art. Pieter Brueghel the Elder painted a large series of works depicting drunken peasants as well as peasants hallucinating under the influence of St. Anthony's fire.[16] His near-contemporary, Hieronymous Bosch, created a number of unique works of nightmarish quality which portray mood- and mind-altering drugs. In the *Garden of Earthly Delights*, many psychoactive botanicals including belladonna, wolfsbane and poppies are seen. *The Seven Deadly Sins* shows alcoholism and drunkenness in both symbolic and realistic form. The *Temptation of St. Anthony* is another depiction of St. Anthony's fire, even though St. Anthony himself was never infected with clavicups.[17]

The lithographer and painter Albrecht Dürer drew depictions of alcoholism which were similar to his etchings of melancholia. The political scientist Niccolo Machiavelli produced a popular play, *Mandragola*, which dealt with the mind-altering effects of the mandrake group.

The great tapestries and sculptures of this time show drunkenness as well as the growing of beer and the fermentation of wine. The accuracy of these depictions shows that the artists were not unfamiliar with drunkenness, hangover or withdrawal. Many excellent tapestries can be found in the vintners' and brewers' guilds of Southern and Northern Europe, respectively.

The authors of this time usually had ambivalent attitudes towards alcohol and other drugs. The dichotomy in the Medieval era between Boccaccio and Chaucer on one hand, and Dante and Bernard on the other, dissolved in the redefining period of the Italian Renaissance. In Benvenuto Cellini's *Autobiography*, the attractions of alcohol are dealt with in a forthright manner.[18] Georgio Vasari's *The Lives of the Most Eminent Painters* is also more of a chronicle than an editorial.[19] This role was assumed by the French balladeer Francoise Villon, whose *Ballades Le Testamente* and his short poem, "In This Whorehouse Where We Do a Roaring Trade," deal with alcoholism in a lusty, earthy, and over-all admiring manner.[20] Alcohol was increasingly viewed as an important element of an exciting lifestyle full of adventure, energy and creativity. The cardinal John Burchard, who served as seneschal to the court of the Borgia Pope Alexander, chronicled the general acceptance of alcoholic excesses and belladonna and mandrake abuse.[21]

As Europe entered the Baroque era, the Italian schools of painting finally began to depict the excesses. Drunkenness became a theme of the great artists of this time, beginning with Michelangelo Caravaggio. The contortion of limbs and the twisting of muscle associated with alcoholic frenzies were duplicated in his experiments with tri-dimensional realism.[22] A host of imitators in the fields of painting and sculpture would reproduce this theme for nearly two centuries.

The rise of Reformation religious sects, especially the Puritans, ironically introduced a rich literature on drug abuse. The only work from that period read today is John Bunyan's *Pilgrim's Progress*.

Quite possibly, the early American writer Washington Irving was influenced by a number of recreational drugs. His "Adantalado of the Seven Cities" appears to be a description written under the influence of opium, whereas his "Headless Horseman" may be derived from an anticholinergic psychosis. The "Legend of the Engulphed Convent," and "Don Juan: a Spectral Research," also may have reflected personal experiments with psychedelic drugs or tales told to him by persons thus affected.[23]

During the Napoleonic Era, it was popular to paint or sculpt allegories of alcohol, opium, and belladonna which, at times, were authentic artistic depictions.

With his work, *Confessions of an English Opium Eater*, James De Quincy became the first person to clinically describe for a popular audience the hallucinations, altered states and withdrawal symptoms associated with opium. The poet Samuel Taylor Coleridge wrote "Xanadu" and "Rime of the Ancient Mariner" under the influence of laudanum tincture of opium.[24] A less mystical description of the destructive effects of opium is provided in George Eliot's *Silas Marner* and *Adam Bede*.

The British explorer Sir Richard Burton was one of the first to describe khat to the European audience. He also translated *Scheherazade* or *The 1001 Arabian Nights* into English, giving an insight into the effects of hashish, opium and khat.

Robert Lewis Stevenson's short morality story, *Dr. Jekyll and Mr. Hyde*, which described a doctor's self-destruction after drug experiments, was translated into every European language. H.G. Wells' *Food of the Gods* and *The Invisible Man* also dealt with the destructive nature of drugs. In both books, his protagonist, like Stevenson's Dr. Jekyll, feels exhilarated and more confident when under the influence, but is eventually destroyed as a result of drug use.[25] A similar theme is addressed in Edgar Allen Poe's "Masque of the Red Death."[26]

Although there is no suggestion that the mystic poet and painter William Blake ever used drugs, there was an antirationalist quality to his works that was later adopted by members of the twentieth century drug culture. Two of his poetic works, *The Book of Los* and *The Book of Uriza*, describe many states which can be experienced under the influence of cocaine, the psychedelics and the opiates.[27] His free-form style of painting was adopted in the nineteenth century, and readopted by the psychedelic painters of the 1960's.

Henri de Toulouse-Lautrec, a French impressionist artist, painted a large series of posters of *fin de siècle* "Rive Gauche" life.[28] His work, especially the depictions of the singer Aristide Bruant and the dancer Jean Avril, were later adopted by purveyors of many mind-altering drugs. Advertisements for Kola Marque and absinthe in France, the cocaine-laden wine vin Mariani in Italy, and for the American-made Hood's sarsaparilla and Dr. Girard's Ginger Brandy so faithfully reproduce Lautrec's style as to be almost-forgeries.[29] These and other medications and beverages which were popular at the time were apt to be mixtures of ginger root and cola nut mixed with cocaine, alcohol, opium, belladonna, asthmador, quinine and strychnine.

In the late eighteenth and early nineteenth centuries, English engraver William Hogarth published *Gin Lane* and *Marriage a la Mode*, a series of lithographs, in protest against the glorification of alcohol, especially as witnessed among the lower and middle classes.[30]

Although marijuana had been discussed in nineteenth century literature and painting, most of these works were generally not significant. The exception is John Tenniel's sly inclusion of his engraving of the marijuana plant, *Cannabis sativa*, in the plates of Lewis Carroll's *Alice in Wonderland* and *Alice Through the Looking Glass*.[31]

FILM, TELEVISION AND THEATER
IN THE TWENTIETH CENTURY

With the dawn of the 20th century, a new art form had developed: the movie. The first depiction of alcoholism was in D.W. Griffith's *The Spoilers*.[32] This 1914 adaptation of the earlier Rex Beech novel dealt with alcoholism in Alaskan pioneers. William S. Hart's classic western, *Hell's Hinges*, made in 1916, followed the alcoholic dissolution of a western minister in a nineteenth century cowboy town.[33]

The German import, Fritz Lang's *Cabinet of Dr. Caligari*, was the first film depiction of altered states.[34] Its special effects were similar to sensory alterations produced by hashish and alcohol.

In 1921, Louis B. Mayer produced the first surviving film version of Robert Lewis Stevenson's *Dr. Jekyll and Mr. Hyde*, a movie which depicted a twisted body and psyche which released unabated evil.[35]

With the decline of the silent movies and the advent of the talkies, the European cinema bloomed with depictions of alcohol as in the German film *Blue Venus* and the Italian film *Rovini*. These themes, however, were not popular among the American audiences. The only memorable film is *Reefer Madness* which was produced in the 1930's. It is worth noting, although not for literary or scholarly content, for there is none. Rather, *Reefer Madness* is seen as a propaganda film which over-exaggerated the detrimental effects of marijuana. Rather than convincing its audience, it made disbelievers of them.

After World War II, Ray Milland's depiction of an alcoholic in *Lost Weekend* is a clinical gem. Withdrawal symptoms, blackouts, and delirium tremens were, for the first time, introduced to the American audience at-large and produced in an artistic, yet clinically correct fashion. In the 1950's, Otto Preminger's equally memorable production of *The Man With The Golden Arm*, faithfully adapted from the Nelson Algren novel, became the first mainstream American movie to depict heroin withdrawal. Frank Sinatra received an Academy Award nomination for his "heart-felt dramatization of the perils of drug abuse," stated the film's publicist.[36] In a later popular film, *Let No Man Write My Epitaph*, Burl Ives portrays a fallen alcoholic judge and James Darren plays a naive early drug abuser.

In 1960's Hollywood, however, the attitude towards drugs slowly changed. The movie *Bob & Carol & Ted & Alice* displayed two suburban couples for whom marijuana use was slightly daring and somewhat off-limits. The same attitude was reflected by society on the other side of the tracks when marijuana was used by a male prostitute in *The Midnight Cowboy*.

This attitude quickly changed. Suddenly marijuana was acceptable and those who opposed it were seen as ridiculous if not despicable. In the movies *Easy Rider* and *Joe*, the heroes mix marijuana, liberal sexual views, pacifism and rejection of materialism into a positive heroic role. Erich Segal's script for the *Yellow Submarine* developed visual and symbolic images associated with the drug culture. Interestingly, at that time the Disney movies *Fantasia* and *Alice and Wonderland* were revived and shown at movie theaters where the air was heavy with marijuana smoke and members of the audience dropped acid through these subjectively transmogrified double features.[37]

Inevitably, counter-reaction set in. The cinematic vehicles which reflected this change were period pieces. The first were Federico Fellini's film version of Titus Petronius Arbiter's *Satyricon* and Robert Altman's western, *McCabe and Mrs. Miller*.[38] Fellini used his typical surrealistic and sometimes psychedelic view of ancient Rome to display an allegorical degeneration that was symbolical of the contemporary drug culture in Italy. In Altman's film, the men of the western town are dissipated by alcohol while Mrs. Miller, the owner of the town's most successful business, a brothel, loses herself in an opium den. The destructive and fatal effects of amphetamine were next explored in Bob Fosse's semi-autobiographical *All That Jazz*. The destructive nature of a mescaline-like psychedelic drug was studied in Paddy Chayersky's *Altered States*.

Television was another new artistic medium of the twentieth century. However, it did not deal seriously with alcoholism or drug abuse on a regular basis. There were single performance plays in such repertory series as Armstrong Circle Theater, U.S. Steel Theater and Chrysler Playhouse. The only television series of the 1950's which dealt with alcoholism was *Topper*. In this series, the alcoholic was a ghost that happened to be a St. Bernard dog.

Several comedians such as Jackie Gleason, Red Skelton and Sid Cesar developed alcoholic characters, but they, like the ghostly St. Bernard, were seen as comedic figures. The later fad of medical shows such as Richard Boone's *Medic*, as well as its imitators, *Ben Casey* and *Dr. Kildare*, dealt with drug abuse in some episodes.

In the 1950's, drug abuse was taboo and alcoholism was not a commercially feasible topic. In the late 1960's and early 1970's, alcohol was dealt with in an eye-winking fashion by the singer-actor, Dean Martin, and similar comedians in variety shows. In the 1980's, the television screen exploded with a number of dramatic and comedic roles dealing with alcoholism and drug addiction.

On Broadway, many of the works of Tennessee Williams, especially *The Rose Tattoo* and *Cat on a Hot Tin Roof*, dealt with alcoholism. Both of these plays were later made into movies. Michael Gazzo's *Hat Full of Rain* gave a realistic depiction of a heroin addict and the corrosive effects the addiction had on his family. In *The Days of Wine and Roses*, a play which was also made into a movie, Jack Lemmon and Lee Remick explore a married couple's alcoholic seduction and the husband's subsequent abandonment of his wife when she cannot recover from the addiction he initiated.

In the 1960's, Broadway's moralistic attitude towards drugs changed dramatically. The agent of this change was a small off-Broadway play *Hair*, written by Gerome Ragni and James Rado. Within *Hair*'s lyrical content, all conventions against drug, sex and frontal nudity were destroyed. *Hair* invaded Broadway, the musical recording industry, Hollywood and community theaters across the United States.[39] In short fashion, there followed the combination of the Bible and drugs in the rock opera, *Godspell*. The rock group The Who released the rock opera, *Tommy*. With its images of acid queens, pinball wizards and pill-pushing quack doctors, *Tommy* continued in the direction that *Hair* had started.

MUSIC OF THE TWENTIETH CENTURY

There was a dichotomy in early twentieth century music. Except for the short-lived success of the "gin singers" during the Prohibition Era, mainstream "white" music did not discuss alcoholism or drug abuse. This, however, was not true of the blues or other musical expressions of black American culture. "St. James Infirmary" and other songs dealt with the despair of addicted men and women.

Marijuana was considered part of the culture of jazz music. Although jazz songs did not express any specific attitudes towards marijuana, jazz musicians were thought to have experimented extensively with this particular drug in the creation and performance of their musical works.

The subject of alcohol was taken up in the 1930's by country and western singers and songwriters. Generally, men would relate the travails of alcoholism. Another small segment of white America heard the anti-alcohol and anti-drug message through newly coined folk songs that were written during the Depression era. The most popular were variants of "Streets of Loredo," except that the victim expires not from a bullet in the chest but from sundry acts of dissolution including alcohol and marijuana.

Most of the show tunes that were sung by white America ignored alcoholism. There were, however, exceptions. Kirk Weill's and Bertolt Brecht's opera *The Rise and Fall of the City of Mahogonny* is the story of a prostitute whose life is spent in a quest for the "next whiskey bar" until she is "bound to die." While black music forthrightly dealt with drug and alcohol addiction, white music rarely mentioned alcohol or other drugs. The rare mention—such as Cole Porter's "I get no kick from cocaine, mere alcohol doesn't thrill me at all"— was usually in passing.[40]

This changed during the psychedelic era of the 1960's. Drugs now became a positive symptom and leitmotif of the post-war generation. Arlo Guthrie was able to commercially extol marijuana in his song, "Alice's Restaurant," and cocaine in his shorter piece, "Coming into Los Angeles."[41] A relatively soft-rock group, The Association, wrote about marijuana as a cure for adolescent angst in "Along Comes Mary." The Beatles scored for psychedelics in "Lucy in the Sky with Diamonds." This was followed by Donovan Leitch's murkily symbolic songs, "Mellow Yellow" and "Sunshine Superman." Finally, a whole genre of songs called acid rock developed, which were meant to be listened to under the influence of psychedelic drugs. One such song was "White Rabbit," which Marty Ballan wrote for his two successive musical groups, The Great Society and Jefferson Airplane.

Although war babies extolled many of the drugs which their parents scorned, they still retained some attitudes of the 1930's and 1940's culture. Alcoholism was still seen as a sign of weakness, as reflected in Ian Anderson's "Aqualung," written for the band Jethro Tull.[42] Heroin was also condemned in Steppenwolf's "Goddamn the Pusher Man."

Inevitably, fatigue and maturity lead to the decline of the Sixties' drug music culture. This decline was further assisted by the drug-related deaths of many pop singers, such as Janis Joplin, Jimi Hendrix, and Cass Elliott.

LITERATURE OF THE TWENTIETH CENTURY

The "lost generation" provided the first great twentieth century exploration of alcoholism. Ernest Hemingway, Thomas Wolfe and Henry Miller all presented alcohol as one of many avenues of alienation.[43,44] The translation of Herman Hesse's book, *Steppenwolf*, subjectively described a cocaine-like drug.[45]

In the 1930's, Aldous Huxley described a tranquilizing substance in *Brave New World*. This substance called "soma" was disturbingly similar to the tranquilizers developed in the 1960's. The "pill for every ill" was taken with the admonition, "a gram instead of a damn."[46] In Huxley's allegorical *After Many A Summer Dies the Swan*, the protagonist is offered immortal life in the form of a pill that has the unfortunate side effect of reducing him to a gorilla-like state.

During this time period, the popular American detective story writer Dashiell Hammett wrote *The Dain Curse*. This popular work dealt with drug abuse and reflected the public's fear and repugnance towards illicit drugs.

After World War II, "polite" novels such as John Marquand's *Women and Thomas Harrow*, dealt with society's rejection of such relatively mild mind-altering drugs such as sleeping pills.[47] The great post-war novels, including Norman Mailer's *The Naked and the Dead*, and John Jones' *The Thin Red Line*, realistically and effectively described alcoholism as a crutch to the victorious American soldier.

During the 1950's, the literary trinity of the beat generation, Lawrence Ferlinghetti, Allen Ginsberg and Jack Kerouac, published a series of books that first presented the liberal attitude in a commercially acceptable artistic form.[48] It was during this time that Nelson Algren wrote the novel *Man With A Golden Arm*, which later became the Otto Preminger film discussed earlier. Within the genre of science fiction, Alfred Bester wrote *The Stars, My Destination*. Whether by intuition or by knowledge of the discovery of LSD by Swiss chemist Alfred Hoffman, Bester used subjective descriptions and unique, oddly spaced typography to convey to the reader the psychedelic state.[49]

In the 1960's, the novelist Ken Kesey published *One Flew Over The Cuckoo's Nest*. This story of an insane asylum dichotomized drugs into the "bad" type prescribed by psychiatrists and the "good" type symbolized by marijuana. Tom Wolfe wrote a journalistic novel entitled *Electric Kool-Aid Acid Test* that described Ken Kesey's adventures.[50] Both were huge successes. The former became an Academy Award-winning movie.

Anthony Burgess scored off Aldous Huxley to write *A Clockwork Orange*, in which drugs, dispensed in milk through the fiberglass breasts of female mannequins, provided a means of social control.[51] At the time *A Clockwork Orange* was produced as a movie, Carlos Castaneda wrote his semi-fictional *Ring of Fire*. In this book, Castaneda is guided by psychedelic drugs into mystical realms by a Mexican Indian holy man.

Whereas Carlos Castaneda sanctified the role of drugs, James Bugliosi tried to develop strong sanctions against their use. This former prosecutor who successfully secured convictions against the Charles Manson gang in California for the murder of Sharon Tate and others, wrote about the role of drugs in creating a cult whose members committed murder at the behest of their charismatic leader. His book, *Helter Skelter*, helped to encourage the public to question the drug culture.

At this time, Aldous Huxley created a new work, *Brave New World, Revisited*. In this book, he adopted a uniquely personal view. While Huxley did not see any difficulty with a personal decision to use drugs, he warned against the potential for social control which these very drugs occasioned.[52]

In the science fiction genre, George Herbert published his six-volume series on *Dune*. In it, a drug termed "spice" and derived from the death of giant worms, is able to give longevity and special mental powers to the users. Spice, however, carries a heavy price: those who use it ultimately are destroyed.[53] In the same genre, Philip Jose Farmer published his seven-volume *World of the Tiers* series over a 20-year period ending in 1995. In this series, he recreates the universes of William Blake. In the sixth and seventh volumes, he reveals that these worlds can be attained by mystics such as Blake, as well as drug addicts living near the edge of psychosis.[1,54]

VISUAL ART OF THE TWENTIETH CENTURY

While the literary and performing arts have continued to illustrate the richly woven tapestry of drug culture in this century, the visual arts have not. Aside from the cubists' flattening perspective pioneered by George Bracque and Pablo Picasso, and the derivative angularity of Tamara de Lempicka, which display the geometricization and flattening found in mescaline-induced visual distortions, little else has been pioneered.[55]

American painters such as George Bellow and George Luks dealt specifically with the effects of alcoholism on their coarsened subjects, though this style did not survive the post-World War II period. The post-war abstractionism, op-art, and pop-art did little to depict the drug culture, although much op-art provided visual toys for drug-abusing viewers. The style of Peter Max and his imitators, deriving from William Blake's roots, recreated the ambiance, attitudes and dress of the drug-supported cultures of the 1960's. It was quickly adapted to album covers, posters, bed spreads, paper plates and other disposable and semi-disposable relics of that era.

Cartooning, however, did continuously address alcoholism and later the effects of drugs. The early cartoons of this century, including *Bringing Up Father* and the *Katzenjammer Kids*, amused readers with the foibles of alcoholic adults. Al Capp's *Lil' Abner* satirically portrayed alcoholics who were addicted to his mythical Dogpatch's distilled concoction, "Kickapoo Joy Juice." The war cartoon *Terry and the Pirates* courageously dealt with alcoholic pilots and opium-addicted victims of the Dragon Lady. In the 60's, the bizarre cartoon style of R. Crumb reflected a generational divide. He portrayed positive attitudes towards drug use in young adults but negative attitudes towards alcoholism in the older generation in his *Zap Comix* and *Fritz The Cat*.

Today as attitudes towards drugs evolve and revolve, societal forces remain in flux. The cable television industry reflects a rejectionist attitude towards drug abuse, whereas broadcasting networks and the movie industry portray a more accepting one.[56] These opposing views may passively represent the split attitudes of a society which has not accepted but not yet rejected the drugs of abuse.

NOTES

1. Giannini AJ. Afterword. In: PJ Farmer (Ed.), Red Orcs Rage. New York: Tor Books, 1992.
2. Xenephon. Oeconomicus. Boston: Little Brown, 1927.
3. Sallust. The Jugurthine War. London: Cox & Wymann, 1963.
4. Dio Cassius C. History of Rome. New York: Troy, 1905.
5. Arbiter TP. Satyricon. Los Angeles: Holloway, 1965.
6. Statue of Gudea, Governor of Lagash. London: British Museum of Art, Acquisition, 1860.
7. Mural in the House of Eqauilus, Ancient Pompeii. Naples, Italy.
8. King CM (Ed.). The Venerable Bede's Ecclesiastical History of England. London: Oxford, 1917.
9. Bonner A. Songs of the Troubadours. New York: Schocken, 1972.
10. Works of St. Bernard of Clairvaux. Indianapolis: Cistercian Fathers, 1970.
11. Crawford R. Plague and Pestilence in Literature and Art. Oxford: Oxford Univ Press, 1914.
12. Alighieri D. Il Comedio Divina. New York: Random House. 1932
13. Boccaccio G. Decameron. New York: Doubleday, 1930.
14. Ward CF (Ed.). The Epistles on the Romance of the Rose. Chicago: Univ Chicago, 1911.
15. The Letters of Abelard and Heloise. London: Moncrieff, 1925.
16. Grauls J. Volkstaal en volskleven in net werk van Pieter Brueghel. Rotterdam: deGroot, 1975.
17. DeTolnay C. Hieronymous Bosch. Baden-Baden: Holle Verlag, 1965.
18. Cellini B. Autobiography. London: MacMillan, 1928.
19. Vasari G. The Lives of the Most Eminent Painters. New York: Heritage, 1967.
20. Villon F. The Legacy, the Testament and other Poems. New York: St. Martin's Press, 1943.
21. Burchard B. Diarun 1548. London: Plessey, 1982.
22. Van Marle R. The Development Italian Schools of Painting. New York: Hacker Art Books, 1970.
23. Neider C. The Complete Tales of Washington Irving. Garden City: Doubleday, 1979.
24. Deutsch B. Poems of Samuel Taylor Coleridge. New York: Thomas Y. Crowell, 1967.

25. Wells HG. Seven Famous Novels. New York: Knopf, 1934.
26. Poe EA. Complete Stories and Poems. New York: Doubleday, 1966.
27. Borges JL, Schiff G. Blake in Heaven and Hell. FMR (American Edition) 1984; **1**:67.
28. Joyant M. Henri de Toulouse-Lautrec. Paris, DeDion, 1927.
29. Lyons AS, Petrucelli, RJ. Medicine - The Illustrated History. New York: Albradale Press, 1978.
30. Hogarth W. Marriage a la Mode. London: Longman, Hurst, Reese & Orme, 1793.
31. Gardner M. Lewis Carroll: The Annotated Alice. New York: Bramhall House, 1960.
32. Griffiths DW. The Spoilers. New York: Selig Polyscope, 1914.
33. Hart WS. Hell's Hinges. Los Angeles: Ince-Triangle, 1916.
34. Lang F. Cabinet of Dr. Caligari. Berlin: Pommer, 1929.
35. Stevenson RL. Dr. Jekyll and Mr. Hyde. Los Angeles: Paramount, 1920.
36. Preminger O. The Man With A Golden Arm. Los Angeles: Paramount, 1956.
37. Culhane J. Walt Disney's Fantasia. New York: Abradale Press, 1983.
38. Altman R. McCabe and Mrs. Miller. Los Angeles: Warner Bros, 1971.
39. Ragni G, Rado J, MacDermot G. Hair. New York: Natoma Productions, 1968.
40. Weill K, Brecht B. The Rise and Fall of The City of Mahogonny. (Aufstig und Fall der Stadt Mahogonny). Berlin: Reinhardt & Piscator, 1930.
41. Guthrie A. Alice's Restaurant. Burbank: Reprise, 1967.
42. Anderson I. Aqualung. London: Chrysalis, 1971.
43. Hemingway E. For Whom the Bell Tolls. New York: Charles Scribner's Sons, 1940.
44. Miller H. Nexus. Paris: Les Editions du Chene, 1960.
45. Hesse H. Steppenwolf. Berlin: S Fischer Verlag, 1929.
46. Huxley A. Brave New World. New York: Harper, 1938.
47. Marquand T. Women and Thomas Harrow. Boston: Little Brown, 1958.
48. Ferlinghetti L. Open Eye, Open Heart. New York: New Directions, 1961.

49. Bester A. The Stars, My Destination. New York: Galaxy Publishing, 1956.
50. Wolfe T. The Electric Kool-Aid Acid Test. New York: Farrar, Straus & Giroux, 1968.
51. Burgess A. A Clockwork Orange. New York: WW Norton, 1963.
52. Huxley A. Brave New World Revisited. New York: Harper Row, 1968.
53. Herbert G. Dune. New York: Ace, 1965.
54. Farmer PJ. More Than Fire. New York: Tor Books, 1993.
55. Marmori G, Abrasino A. Tamara: Painting the beaumonde. FMR (English Edition). 1986;18:67-89.
56. Goldberg R, Goldberg GJ. Citizen Turner. New York: Harcourt, Brace & Co. 1995.

APPENDIX B

GUIDE TO STREET NAMES
OF DRUGS OF ABUSE

For the reader's convenience, the current street names for the drugs of abuse discussed in this volume are listed below.

STREET NAME	CHEMICAL NAME	CLASS
A		
Absinthe	Tincture of wormwood	Ethanol
Acapulco gold	Marijuana	Marijuana
Ace	Barbiturate	Sedative-Hypnotic
Ace	Marijuana	Marijuana
Acid	Lysergic acid	Psychedelic
Adam	Methylenedioxymethamphetimine	Psychedelic
African black	Marijuana	Marijuana
All-American	Methamphetamine	Sympathomimetic
AMT	Dimethyltryptamine	Psychedelic
Amy	Amyl nitrite	Volatile
Angel dust	Phencyclidine	Dissociative
Annulene	Benzene	Volatile
Asthma weed	Asthmador	Anticholinergic
Aztec	Psilocybin	Psychedelic
B		
Bad acid	Lysergic acid with strychnine	Psychedelic
Bad seed	Mescaline	Psychedelic
Bail	Marijuana	Marijuana
Bams	Meprobamate	Sedative-Hypnotic
Banana	Barbiturate	Sedative-Hypnotic
Banana split	Barbiturate	Sedative-Hypnotic
Bang	Marijuana	Marijuana
Barbs	Barbiturate	Barbiturate
Base	Cocaine	Sympathomimetic
Baseball	Crack cocaine	Cocaine
Base-rock	Crack cocaine	Cocaine
Batu	Methamphetamine/crystalline	Sympathomimetic
Belladonna	Atropine	Anticholinergic
Bennies	Amphetamine	Sympathomimetic
B hang	Marijuana (leaves & shoots)	Marijuana
Black beauties	Amphetamine	Sympathomimetic

B *(continued)*

Black rose	Oil of cloves	Psychedelic (spurious)
Bladder pod	Asthmador	Anticholinergic
Blotter	Lysergic acid	Psychedelic
Blotter Acid	Lysergic acid	Psychedelic
Blow	Cocaine	Sympathomimetic
Blow	Marijuana	Marijuana
Blue and White	Glutethimide	Sedative-Hypnotic
Blue Bird	Barbiturate	Sedative-Hypnotic
Blue cap	Mescaline	Psychedelic
Blue cardinal	Asthmador	Anticholinergic
Blue cheer	Lysergic acid	Amphetamine
Blue devil	Barbiturate	Sedative-Hypnotic
Blue racers	Barbiturate	Sedative-Hypnotic
Blue velvet	Tripelennamine with codeine	Anticholinergic/Opiate
Blues	Barbiturate	Sympathomimetic
Bolivian	Cocaine	Sympathomimetic
Bomber	Marijuana	Marijuana
Bombita	Amphetamine	Sympathomimetic
Boo	Marijuana	Marijuana
Boone's farm	Cheap wine	Ethanol
Boy-Girl	Cocaine/Heroin	Sympathomimetic/Opiate
Bright eyes	Asthmador	Anticholinergic
Brown slime	Nutmeg	Psychedelic
B.T.-72s	Phenylpropanolamine	Sympathomimetic
Bull	Malt liquor	Alcohol
Businessman's lunch	Dimethyltryptamine	Psychedelic
Buster Brown	Phencyclidine	Dissociative
Button	Mescaline	Psychedelic

C

C	Cocaine	Sympathomimetic
Cactus	Mescaline	Psychedelic
California sunshine	Lysergic acid	Psychedelic
Candy	Cocaine	Sympathomimetic
Cannabis	Marijuana	Marijuana
Caramel delights	Heroin tar	Opiate
Carbon oil	Benzene	Volatile
Cathouse drops	Amyl nitrite	Volatile
CB	Glutethimide	Sedative-Hypnotic
Charas	Hashish	Opiate
Chiba	Marijuana	Marijuana
Chief	Mescaline	Psychedelic
China cat	Heroin	Opiate
China white	Methamphetamine, crystalline	Sympathomimetic
Christmas trees	Amphetamine	Sympathomimetic
Ciba	Glutethimide	Sedative-Hypnotic
Clocks	Atropine	Anticholinergic
Coke	Cocaine	Sympathomimetic
Colt .45	Malt liquor	Alcohol

C *(continued)*

Copilot	Phenylpropanolamine	Sympathomimetic
Christina	Methamphetamine, crystalline	Sympathomimetic
Crack	Crack cocaine	Sympathomimetic
Crank	Methamphetamine, crystalline	Sympathomimetic
Crystal	Methamphetamine, crystalline	Sympathomimetic
Crystal meth	Methamphetamine, crystalline	Sympathomimetic
Cube	Lysergic acid	Psychedelic

D

Deadly nightshade	Atropine-containing mushroom	Anticholinergic
Deca	Testosterone	Steroid
Deer Bull	Nandrolone	Steroid
Depo	Testosterone	Steroid
Dexies	Amphetamine	Sympathomimetic
DMT	Dimethyltryptamine	Psychedelic
Dolphin	Methadone	Opiate
DOM	Dimethoxymethylamphetamine	Psychedelic
Doobie	Marijuana	Marijuana
Dope	Marijuana	Marijuana
Downs	Barbiturate	Sedative-Hypnotic
Dudley-do-right	Ethanol, distilled	Ethanol
Dust	Cocaine	Sympathomimetic
Dust	Opiate	Opiate
Dust	Phencyclidine	Dissociative
Dyne-o-mite	Heroin	Opiate

E

Easter bunnies	Methyprylon	Sedative-hypnotic
Ecstacy	Methylenedioxymethamphetamine	Psychedelic
Eight ball	Crack cocaine	Cocaine
Eve	Free-base cocaine	Sympathomimetic
Express	Amphetamine	Sympathomimetic

F

F-40S	Barbiturate	Sedative-Hypnotic
Flake	Cocaine	Sympathomimetic
Flying saucer	Morning glory seed	Psychedelic
Free-base	Cocaine	Sympathomimetic
Freeze	Cocaine	Sympathomimetic
French blues	Amphetamine/Barbiturate	Sympathomimetic/ Sedative-Hypnotic

G

Gag root	Asthmador	Anticholinergic
Ganja	Marijuana resin	Marijuana
Geezer	Opiate	Opiate
Gin	Cocaine	Cocaine
Gold	Marijuana	Marijuana
Gold dust	Cocaine	Sympathomimetic

G *(continued)*

Gong	Marijuana	Marijuana
Gong	Opium	Opiate
Goofball	Barbiturate	Sedative-Hypnotic
Gram	Hashish	Marijuana
Grass	Marijuana	Marijuana
Greenie	Ethchlorvynol	Sedative-Hypnotic
Greens	Chloral hydrate	Alcohol

H

H	Heroin	Opiate
H & C	Opiate/Cocaine	Sympathomimetic
Halloweens	Barbiturate	Sedative-Hypnotic
Happy Dust	Cocaine	Sympathomimetic
Harrary	Khat	Sympathomimetic
Hash	Hashish	Marijuana
Hay	Marijuana	Marijuana
Hearts	Amphetamine	Sympathomimetic
Heavenly Blues	Morning glory seeds	Psychedelic
Hemp	Marijuana	Marijuana
Herb	Marijuana	Marijuana
High C	Cocaine	Sympathomimetic
Highmaster	Marijuana	Marijuana
Hip	Opiate	Opiate
Hocus	Opiate	Opiate
Hog	Phencyclidine	Dissociative
Hog physic	Asthmador	Anticholinergic
Honalee	Heroin	Opiate
Horse	Heroin	Opiate

I

Ice	Methamphetamine, Crystalline	Sympathomimetic
Indian tobacco	Asthmador	Anticholinergic
Island sunshine	Marijuana	Marijuana

J

Java	Caffeine	Sympathomimetic
Jelly beans	Chloral hydrate	Alcohol
Jimson weed	Atropine	Anticholinergic
Johnny Binder	Crack cocaine	Sympathomimetic
Joint	Marijuana	Marijuana
Juju bee's	Chloral hydrate	Alcohol

K

Kaui electric	Marijuana	Marijuana
Keefer	Hashish	Hashish
Keets	Ketamine	Dissociative
Kinnikinnik	Asthmador	Anticholinergic
Knockout drops	Chloral hydrate	Alcohol
Kona gold	Marijuana	Marijuana
Krystal	Phencyclidine	Dissociative
Krystal joint	Phencyclidine/Marijuana	Dissociative/Marijuana

L

Laudanum	Mixture of opium, ethanol .... & saffron	Opiate/ethanol
Leaf	Khat	Sympathomimetic
Leaf	Marijuana	Sympathomimetic
Lebanese Blonde ...	Marijuana	Marijuana
Lemons	Methaqualone	Sedative-Hypnotic
Lid	Marijuana	Marijuana
Lilies	Propoxyphene	Opiate
Locker room	Isobutyl nitrite	Volatile
Loco	Marijuana	Marijuana
Loco weed	Atropine	Anticholinergic
Louisiana belle	Asthmador	Anticholinergic
Lou-Lou	Asthmador	Anticholinergic
Love Drug	Methylenedioxymethamphetamine ..	Psychedelic
Low Belia	Asthmador	Anticholinergic
Ludes	Methaqualone	Sedative-Hypnotic
Luminal	Barbiturate	Sedative-Hypnotic

M

Mad dog	Cheap wine	Alcohol
Magic	Dimethoxymethylamphetamine	Sympathomimetic
Magic Mushroom ...	Psilocybin	Psychedelic
Marduff	Khat	Sympathomimetic
Mary Jane	Marijuana	Marijuana
Mary Juanita	Marijuana	Marijuana
Mary Warren	Marijuana	Marijuana
Maui Wowie	Marijuana	Marijuana
Mesc	Mescaline	Psychedelic
Meth	Methadone	Opiate
Meth	Methamphetamine	Sympathomimetic
Mex	Mescaline	Psychedelic
Mexican Airline	Marijuana	Marijuana
Mexican Horse	Heroin	Opiate
Michael Finnegan ...	Chloral hydrate/ethanol	Alcohol
Mickey Finn	Chloral hydrate/ethanol	Alcohol
Mickey Mouse	Lysergic acid	Psychedelic
Mist	Phencyclidine	Dissociative
Mister Green Jeans ..	Ethchlorvinyl	Sedative-Hypnotic
Mister Natural	Lysergic acid	Psychedelic

M *(continued)*

Monkey dust	Heroin	Opiate
Mooch	Heroin	Opiate
Moonshine	Ethanol	Alcohol
Morp	Morphine	Opiate
Motor oil-20	Caffeine	Sympathomimetic
Mountain dew	Ethanol, distilled	Alcohol
Muggles	Marijuana	Marijuana
Muscle man	Steroid	Steroid

N

Naturals	Barbiturate	Barbiturate
Nemmies	Barbiturate	Sedative-Hypnotic
Nightmare blues	Barbiturate	Sedative-Hypnotic
Nose candy	Cocaine	Sympathomimetic
Night train	Cheap fortified wine	Alcohol

O

Oil	Hashish	Hashish
O.J.	Heroin/Marijuana	Opiate/Marijuana
Orange Barrel	Methadone	Opiate
Orange Sunshine	Lysergic acid	Psychedelic
Oranges	Amphetamine	Sympathomimetic
Oreos	Ethenelone	Steroid
Ozoline	Lysergic acid	Psychedelic

P

Panama Red	Marijuana	Marijuana
Panatella	Marijuana	Marijuana
Paste	Coca paste	Cocaine
PCP	Phencyclidine	Dissociative
Peace pill	Phencyclidine	Dissociative
Peanut	Barbiturate	Barbiturate
Pearl	Amyl nitrite	Volatile
Pearly gates	Morning glory seeds	Psychedelic
Pentothal	Barbiturate	Sedative-hypnotic
Perks	Percodan	Opiate
Peruvian	Cocaine	Sympathomimetic
Phene	Benzene	Volatile
Peyote	Mescaline	Psychedelic
Pickle	Ethchlorvinyl	Sedative-Hypnotic
Pinks	Barbiturate	Sedative-Hypnotic
Pin wheels	Opium or Heroin	Opiate
Pin Yee	Opium	Opiate
P.J.'s	Metronidazole/ethanol	Alcohol
Popper	Amyl nitrite	Volatile
Porkers	Phencyclidine	Dissociative
Pot	Marijuana	Marijuana
Puke weed	Asthmador	Anticholinergic
Puma Gold	Marijuana	Marijuana

P *(continued)*

Pumpkin seeds	Alprazolam	Benzodiazepine
Purps	Barbiturate	Barbiturate
Purple microdot	Lysergic acid	Psychedelic
Purple passion	Psilocybin	Psychedelic
Pussy juice	Metronidazole/ethanol	Alcohol

Q

Quaaludes	Methaqualone	Dissociative

R

Rambo	Crack cocaine	Cocaine
Red Bird	Phenylpropanolamine	Sympathomimetic
Red Devils	Phenylpropanolamine	Sympathomimetic
Red lobelia	Asthmador	Anticholinergic
Reds	Phenylpropanolamine	Sympathomimetic
Reefer	Marijuana	Marijuana
Roach	Marijuana	Marijuana
Roach-19	Methyprylon	Sedative-Hypnotic
Roaches	Diazepam	Benzodiazepine
Rock	Crack cocaine	Sympathomimetic
Rocket fuel	Phencyclidine	Dissociative
Rope	Hashish	Marijuana
Rosie	Cheap wine	Ethanol
Roxanne	Crack cocaine	Cocaine

S

Sand	Nutmeg	Psychedelic
Satan's trumpet	Atropine	Anticholinergic
Scrap iron	Ethanol, denatured	Alcohol
Scarlet lobelia	Asthmador	Anticholinergic
Seeds	Morning glory seeds	Psychedelic
Serenity, tranquility peace	"Designer" fentanyl	Sympathomimetic
Seven fourteen	Methaqualone	Sedative-Hypnotic
Shabu	Methamphetamine	Sympathomimetic
Six pack	Fentanyl	Opiate
Skag	Heroin	Opiate
Smack	Heroin	Opiate
Smash	Hashish	Hashish
Snappers	Amyl nitrite	Volatile
Snow	Cocaine	Sympathomimetic
Snuff	Heroin/Marijuana	Opiate
Snuff	Phencyclidine/Tobacco	Phencyclidine
Soapers	Methaqualone	Sedative-Hypnotic
Somalian	Khat	Sympathomimetic
Speed	Amphetamine	Sympathomimetic
Speed ball	Amphetamine/Heroin	Sympathomimetic/Opiate
Speed ball	Cocaine/Opiate	Cocaine/Opiate

S *(continued)*

Space base	Phencyclidine/Crack cocaine	Dissociative
Stick	Marijuana	Marijuana
STP	"Designer" fentanyl	Sympathomimetic
Sweatsock	Isobutyl nitrite	Volatile

T

Tea	Marijuana	Marijuana
Teriyaki	Heroin	Opiate
THC	Tetrahydrocannabinol	Marijuana
THP	Trihexyphenidyl	Anticholinergic
Thunderbird	Cheap wine	Alcohol
Toke	Marijuana	Marijuana
Toot	Cocaine	Sympathomimetic
Tootsie roll	Heroin tar	Opiate
Tranks	Benzodiazapine	Benzodiazepine
Trixies	Trihexyphenidyl	Anticholinergic
Truth Serum	Sodium pentothal	Barbiturate
T's and blues	Pentazocine/Tripelennamine	Opiate/Antihistamine
Tuinal	Barbiturate	Barbiturate
Twenty-twenty	Cheap wine	Alcohol
Twist	Marijuana	Marijuana

U

Ups	Amphetamine	Sympathomimetic

V

Vapors	Glue	Volatile

W

Weed	Marijuana	Marijuana
White cross	Amphetamine	Sympathomimetic
White cross	Methamphetamine	Sympathomimetic
White crystal	Cocaine	Cocaine
White girl	Cocaine	Cocaine
White lemon	Methaqualone	Sympathomimetic
White mole	Amphetamine	Sympathomimetic
White lightning	Ethanol, distilled	Alcohol
Whites	Amphetamine	Amphetamine
White powder	Cocaine	Sympathomimetic
Window pane	Lysergic Acid	Psychedelic
Winston	Stanozolol	Steroid

X

Xanadu	Opium tea (poppy seed infusion)	Opiate
XTC	Methylenedioxymethamphetamine	Psychedelic

Y

Yellow Jackets . . . . . Nembutal . . . . Barbiturate
Yellow Zonker . . . . . . Nembutal . . . . Barbiturate
Yen Shee . . . . Opium . . . . Opiate

Z

Zonker . . . . Nembutal . . . . Barbiturate

INDEX